# NURSING84 BOOKS™

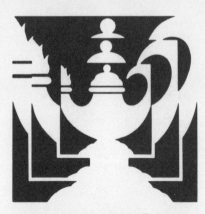

**NURSING NOW™ SERIES**
Shock
Hypertension
Drug Interactions
Cardiac Crises
Respiratory Emergencies

**NURSING PHOTOBOOK™ SERIES**
Providing Respiratory Care
Managing I.V. Therapy
Dealing with Emergencies
Giving Medications
Assessing Your Patients
Using Monitors
Providing Early Mobility
Giving Cardiac Care
Performing GI Procedures
Implementing Urologic Procedures
Controlling Infection
Ensuring Intensive Care
Coping with Neurologic Disorders
Caring for Surgical Patients
Working with Orthopedic Patients
Nursing Pediatric Patients
Helping Geriatric Patients
Attending Ob/Gyn Patients
Aiding Ambulatory Patients
Carrying Out Special Procedures

*Nursing84* DRUG HANDBOOK™

**NURSE'S CLINICAL LIBRARY™**
Cardiovascular Disorders
Respiratory Disorders
Endocrine Disorders
Neurologic Disorders
Renal and Urologic Disorders

**NEW NURSING SKILLBOOK™ SERIES**
Giving Emergency Care Competently
Monitoring Fluid and Electrolytes Precisely
Assessing Vital Functions Accurately
Coping with Neurologic Problems Proficiently
Reading EKGs Correctly
Combatting Cardiovascular Diseases Skillfully
Nursing Critically Ill Patients Confidently

**NURSE'S REFERENCE LIBRARY® SERIES**
Diseases
Diagnostics
Drugs
Assessment
Procedures
Definitions
Practices

# HYPERTENSION

*NURSING84* BOOKS™
SPRINGHOUSE CORPORATION
SPRINGHOUSE, PENNSYLVANIA

# NURSING NOW™ SERIES

EDITORIAL PROJECT DIRECTOR
**Jean Robinson**

CLINICAL DIRECTOR
**Barbara McVan, RN**

ART DIRECTOR
**Lisa A. Gilde**

EDITORIAL MANAGER
**Susan R. Williams**

STAFF FOR THIS VOLUME
BOOK EDITOR
**Katherine W. Carey**

ASSOCIATE EDITORS
**Holly A. Burdick**
**June F. Gomez**
**Deborah Carey Lyons**

CONTRIBUTING EDITOR
**Patricia R. Urosevich**

CLINICAL EDITORS
**Leah A. Gabriel, RN, BSN, MSN**
**Alice R. Perkins, RN, BSN, CCRN**

SENIOR DESIGNER
**Scott M. Stephens**

PRODUCTION COORDINATOR
**Susan Powell-Mishler**

COPY SUPERVISOR
**David R. Moreau**

COPY EDITORS
**Diane M. Labus**
**Jo Lennon**

CONTRIBUTING COPY EDITORS
**Susan Baumann**    **David Jones**
**Reni Fetterolf**    **Doris Weinstock**
**Max A. Fogel**

EDITORIAL ASSISTANTS
**Ellen Johnson**
**Cynthia A. O'Connell**

ART PRODUCTION MANAGER
**Robert Perry**

ARTISTS
**Donald G. Knauss**  **Craig Siman**
**Sandra Sanders**    **Louise Stamper**
**Thom Staudenmayer**

TYPOGRAPHY MANAGER
**David C. Kosten**

TYPOGRAPHY ASSISTANTS
**Janice Haber**      **Diane Paluba**
**Ethel Halle**       **Nancy Wirs**

SENIOR PRODUCTION MANAGER
**Deborah C. Meiris**

PRODUCTION MANAGER
**Wilbur D. Davidson**

PRODUCTION ASSISTANT
**Robin M. Miles**

ILLUSTRATORS
**Michael Adams**     **Robert Jackson**
**Jean Gardner**      **Bob Jones**

PHOTOGRAPHER
**Paul A. Cohen**

COVER PHOTO
**Photographic Illustrations**

CLINICAL CONSULTANTS
FOR THIS VOLUME
**Betty Glenn Harris, RN, PhD**
Assistant Professor, Undergraduate
  Obstetrics, Graduate Nursing
  Theory, University of North
  Carolina School of Nursing,
  Chapel Hill

**Celestine B. Mason, RN, BSN, MA**
Associate Professor, Advanced
  Medical-Surgical Nursing, Pacific
  Lutheran University, Tacoma,
  Wash.

**David M. Rodgers, MD**
Clinical Assistant Professor, Medical
  College of Pennsylvania;
  Cardiologist, Chestnut Hill
  Hospital, Philadelphia

Library of Congress
Cataloging in Publication Data

Main entry under title:
Hypertension.

  (Nursing now series)
  "Nursing 84 books."
  Bibliography: p.
  Includes index.
  1. Hypertension—Nursing.      I. Springhouse
Corporation.    II. Series.    [DNLM:
1. Hypertension—Nursing.     WY 152.5 H9975]
RC685.H8H7675   1984   610.73'691   84-1315
ISBN 0-916730-77-8

# CONTENTS

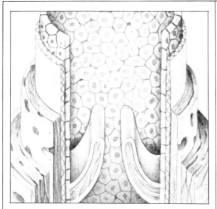

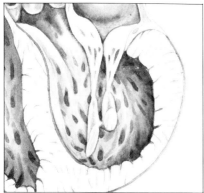

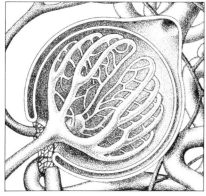

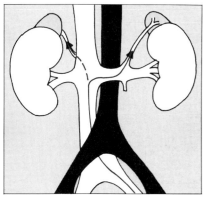

## UNDERSTANDING HYPERTENSION
CELESTINE B. MASON, RN, BSN, MA

## ASSESSING YOUR PATIENT
BETH PULLIAM, RN, BSN, MSN

## MANAGING HYPERTENSION
PATRICIA A. PAYNE, RN-C, MN, FNP

## DEALING WITH SPECIAL PROBLEMS
LINDA Y. ROBERTS, RN
LEAH A. GABRIEL, RN, BSN, MSN
BARBARA McVAN, RN

# CONTRIBUTORS

At the time of publication, these contributors held the following positions:

**Betty Glenn Harris,** an assistant professor at the University of North Carolina School of Nursing in Chapel Hill, teaches undergraduate obstetrics and graduate nursing theory. Ms. Harris received her BSN and MSN degrees from the University of Alabama in Tuscaloosa. She earned her PhD in medical sociology with an emphasis in sociology of the family at North Carolina State University in Raleigh. Ms. Harris is a member of the American Nurses' Association and the American Society for Psychoprophylaxis in Obstetrics, and is president of the Alpha-Alpha chapter of Sigma Theta Tau.

**Celestine B. Mason,** an associate professor at Pacific Lutheran University at Tacoma, Washington, taught advanced medical/surgical and critical care nursing. Ms. Mason received her BSN degree from the Catholic University of America in Washington, D.C., and her MA degree from Pacific Lutheran University. She's currently working toward a degree in law at the University of Puget Sound, Tacoma, Washington.

**Patricia A. Payne** is a nurse practitioner at the Veterans Administration Medical Center in Seattle, Washington. Ms. Payne, who's a member of Sigma Theta Tau, earned her MN degree and her Family Nurse Practitioner certificate at the University of Washington in Seattle.

**Beth Pulliam** is a clinical nurse specialist at the Specialized Center of Research in Hypertension at Vanderbilt University Medical Center in Nashville, Tennessee. She received her BSN degree from Eastern Kentucky University in Richmond, and her MSN degree from Vanderbilt University.

**Linda Y. Roberts** is an administrator at the Heritage Home Health/Heritage Hospice in Bristol, New Hampshire. She received her AAS degree from Mercer County Community College in Trenton, New Jersey. She serves on the boards of the Hospice Affiliates of New Hampshire, the New Hampshire League of Nursing, and the New Hampshire American Cancer Society.

**David M. Rodgers** is a clinical assistant professor at the Medical College of Pennsylvania and an attending cardiologist at Chestnut Hill Hospital, both in Philadelphia. Dr. Rodgers received his BS degree from Pennsylvania State University in University Park and his MD from Jefferson Medical College in Philadelphia.

# INTRODUCTION

The facts about cardiovascular disease (CVD) and hypertension are startling. Consider these points:
• According to the American Heart Association, CVD is the leading cause of death in the United States. Each year, it claims almost as many lives as the other four leading causes of death combined: cancer, accidents, chronic obstructive pulmonary disease, and pneumonia.
• Elevated blood pressure (either systolic or diastolic) is directly related to the development of CVD.
• An estimated 37,330,000 adults have hypertension.

Grim statistics. But the full picture is considerably more encouraging. The American Heart Association also reports that since 1968, deaths from CVD have steadily declined—*despite* rising population and increasing average age.

Why the turnaround? One factor stands out—a concerted effort by the nursing and medical professions to educate the public about hypertension and CVD. And this effort has paid off dramatically. In 1973, more than 1,000,000 Americans died of CVD. In 1978, the figure dropped to 962,000. Today, the downward trend continues.

The conclusion is unavoidable. CVD is a controllable—and perhaps preventable—condition. As you'll learn in this book, hypertension management plays a major part in CVD control.

Where do you fit in? As a nurse, you have daily contact with patients who needlessly risk their lives by ignoring their hypertension. You're in an ideal position to help them minimize the risk.

That's why we feel so strongly about this book. Hypertension is truly a killer—but it's a killer that can be stopped by effective intervention. Few conditions, in fact, provide such opportunity for preventive care.

We've developed this book to help you learn what you need to know about hypertension. In the first section, we discuss the disease's pathophysiology, including its often mysterious causes and potentially devastating effects on blood vessels and organs.

The next two sections focus on your role in assessing and managing the condition. You'll see how to identify a hypertensive patient and assess the severity of his condition. Then, you'll learn about the treatment options available, ranging from nonpharmacologic approaches to drug therapy.

In the final section, you'll find in-depth information about hypertensive crisis, including how to quickly—and safely—lower blood pressure during this emergency. You'll also learn more about several common causes of secondary hypertension and hemorrhagic stroke, a possible complication of hypertension. The book's final pages focus on special considerations for pediatric and geriatric patients who have hypertension.

Throughout this book, we've provided many reproducible patient-teaching aids, because we believe that the battle against hypertension begins with education. Without your patient's informed cooperation, any therapeutic regimen will fail—and the disease will continue to run its destructive course.

Without question, hypertension presents a challenge to your nursing skills. But after you've studied this book, we think you'll feel well prepared to meet it.

Barbara McVan RN

Clinical Director

# UNDERSTANDING HYPERTENSION

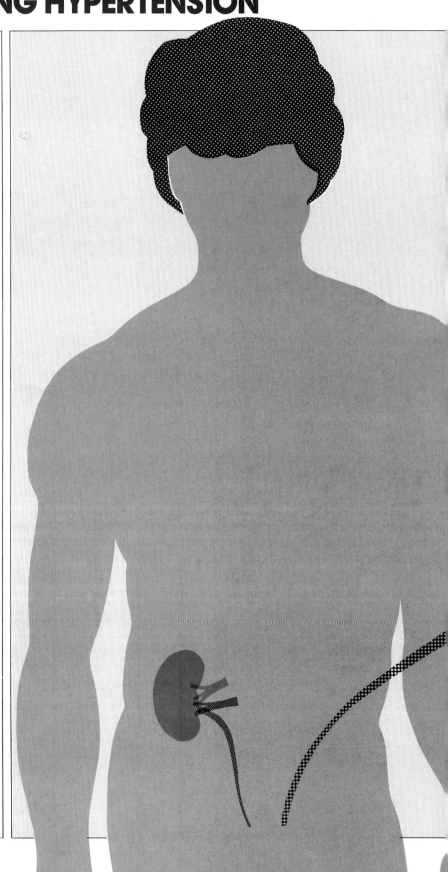

**A**lthough hypertension is a dangerous disease, most cases can be controlled with appropriate therapy. But for therapy to be effective, the patient's compliance is essential. Before he'll comply, he must understand the facts about hypertension: what it is, how it affects his health, and how to control it.

Teaching your patient what he needs to know is a big part of your job. But before you begin, make sure you thoroughly understand this complex disease yourself. This section provides the information you need.

First, we review normal blood pressure regulation, including details on how neuroendocrine hormones contribute to blood pressure stability. Then, we detail the pathophysiology of both primary (essential) and secondary hypertension. With this background, you can better understand hypertension's destructive course and its potentially devastating effects on blood vessels and vital organs.

Armed with the information on these pages, you can help your patient understand why his condition is so serious—and why he must take steps to guard against hypertension's long-term effects.

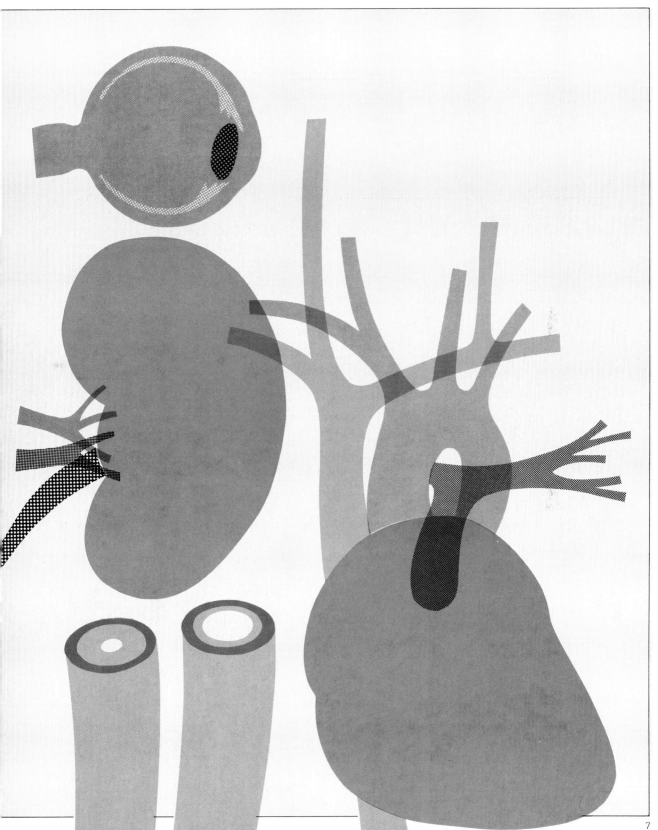

# BLOOD PRESSURE BASICS

## TEACHING YOUR PATIENT THE BASICS

Imagine for a moment that you're talking to a patient who's just learned that he's hypertensive. The news comes as a surprise to him, since he hasn't yet experienced any symptoms. "I have high blood pressure?" he says to you. "What does that mean—do I have too much blood?"

To you, the answer's simple. "No," you might say. "You have the right amount of blood; it just exerts too much pressure against your blood vessel walls."

But to your patient, your simple reply may be mystifying. Remember, he's probably unfamiliar with the basics of anatomy and physiology. What seems like a simple, clear explanation to you may leave *him* more confused than ever.

As a nurse, you'll help oversee your hypertensive patient's treatment, including dietary changes, stress reduction, exercise, and drug therapy. But your biggest challenge is patient teaching.

Think about it. Your patient has a condition that jeopardizes his health—yet he feels fine. Successful treatment may require a major life-style change. And, if drug therapy is indicated, unpleasant side effects may make the treatment seem worse than the disease.

Throughout this book, we'll explore ways you can encourage your patient to comply with treatment. Let's begin by examining a few misconceptions your patient may have about hypertension. The following dialogue suggests questions he may have and how you can answer them in terms he can understand. Also consider using the illustrations on the next few pages to help clarify your points.

**Q:** *The doctor says I have hypertension. That means I'm under a lot of stress and strain, right?*
**A:** Not really, although stress may be a contributing factor. Actually the word *hypertension* is just another name for blood pressure that's too high.

---

*Your patient may have a hard time understanding your concern about his condition—and why his cooperation is essential to a healthy future.*

---

**Q:** *OK, I guess I'm not sure what you mean by blood pressure. Can you explain?*
**A:** To answer your question, I have to start with the heart. The heart pumps blood through blood vessels called arteries. As the blood travels through the arteries, it exerts pressure against the artery walls. That's all blood pressure is—and everyone has it.

You may hear the doctor or me use words like *systolic* and *diastolic* pressure. Systolic pressure is blood pressure when the heart contracts or beats; diastolic pressure is blood pressure between beats, when the heart momentarily relaxes.

**Q:** *Does blood pressure stay the same all the time?*
**A:** No, it goes up and down all day, depending on what you're doing. If you run, for example, it goes up. But when you relax, it should return to a lower level.

In your case, this doesn't happen. Your blood pressure stays too high all the time, even when you're relaxed.

**Q:** *Why does that happen?*
**A:** Although no one knows exactly why, your arteries are under more pressure than they

should be. This means that the force of the blood flowing through the arteries creates a higher pressure.

**Q:** *But I feel fine. Is that unusual?*
**A:** Not at all—and that's why high blood pressure is so dangerous. You can't feel it. But with time, it can damage the blood vessels in your heart, brain, kidneys, and eyes. Eventually, all this pressure can lead to heart attack, stroke, kidney damage, or impaired vision.

**Q:** *What can I do about it?*
**A:** Although we can't *cure* high blood pressure, we can *control* it—with your help. Your doctor and I will help you develop a plan that includes regular checkups, diet changes, exercise, and perhaps medication. By reducing your blood pressure to a safe level and keeping it there, you can avoid injury to body organs.

**Q:** *I don't like to take pills. If I need medicine, how long will I have to take it?*
**A:** For as long as the doctor directs—possibly the rest of your life. To keep your blood pressure under control, you must continue to take your medicine even if you feel fine. Otherwise, your blood pressure will rise again to a dangerous level.

High blood pressure's a dangerous disease. But by following the plan we come up with, you can lead a long, normal life.

## BLOOD VESSELS: A CLOSER LOOK

Vein

Artery

The artery's thick muscle layer helps it withstand high pressure. Because a vein withstands less pressure than an artery, its walls are thinner and more compliant. In the illustration at left, note the vein's valve, which prevents blood backflow.

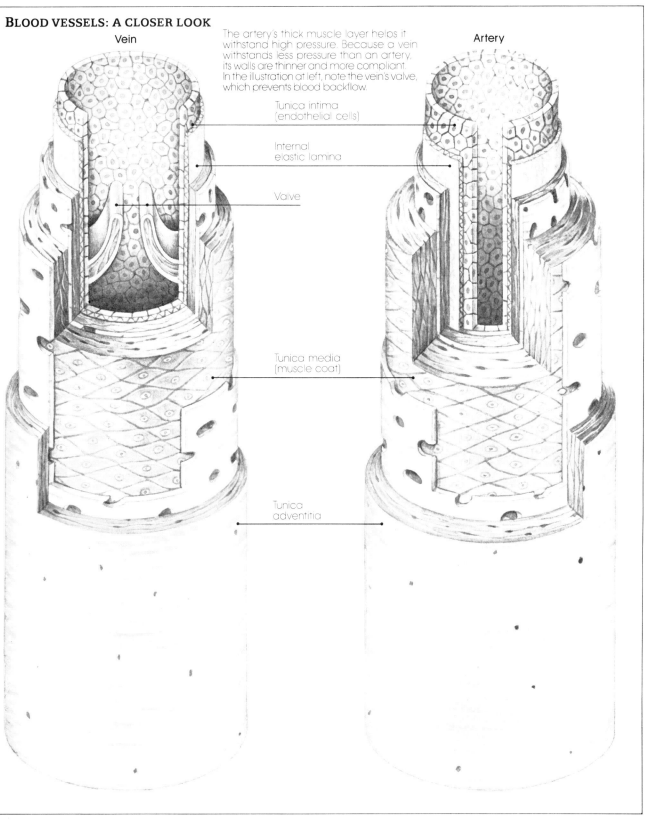

Tunica intima (endothelial cells)

Internal elastic lamina

Valve

Tunica media (muscle coat)

Tunica adventitia

# BLOOD PRESSURE BASICS

## REGULATING BLOOD PRESSURE

Your patient doesn't need to know the complex physiology underlying hypertension. But in order for you to explain the disease in terms he can understand, your own knowledge must be more detailed. Read the following as a quick review of the basics.

**Maintaining homeostasis.** Blood pressure rises and falls—almost from moment to moment—in response to such internal and external influences as physical or emotional stress, temperature changes, drugs, and the body's metabolic needs.

These factors interact to keep blood pressure within safe limits:
• cardiac output. An increase in heart rate or stroke volume raises output and increases blood pressure.
• blood volume. The body must compensate for blood loss to maintain blood pressure.
• blood viscosity. Normally, blood viscosity changes very little; this factor becomes important only in certain abnormal conditions, such as hemorrhage, excessive plasma loss, or severe anemia.
• arterial wall elasticity. Keep in mind that while systolic blood pressure reflects the force of the heart's contractions, diastolic blood pressure reflects the arterial walls' ability to rebound during diastole, when the heart's at rest. Diastolic hypertension reflects the arteries' smaller lumens and thicker walls.
• peripheral resistance (the friction between blood and peripheral vessel walls). A rise in peripheral resistance from increased blood viscosity or loss of arterial wall elasticity or caliber (from arteriosclerosis or vessel constriction) raises blood pressure.

Because blood volume and peripheral resistance are particularly significant in hypertension,

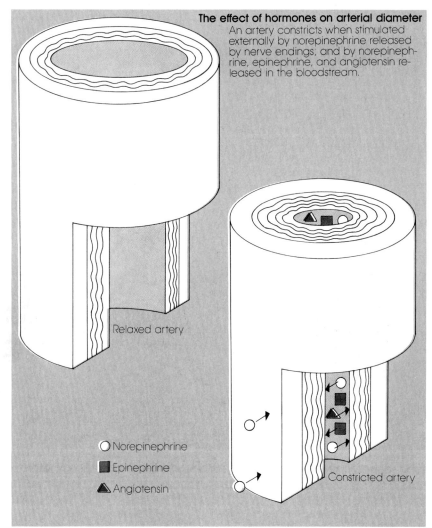

**The effect of hormones on arterial diameter**
An artery constricts when stimulated externally by norepinephrine released by nerve endings; and by norepinephrine, epinephrine, and angiotensin released in the bloodstream.

Relaxed artery

○ Norepinephrine
■ Epinephrine
▲ Angiotensin

Constricted artery

let's take a closer look at these two factors.

**Blood volume.** The kidneys help maintain a stable blood pressure by regulating blood volume. Let's say, for example, that blood pressure drops below normal. To improve blood volume and boost blood pressure, the kidneys conserve sodium and water. On the other hand, if blood pressure suddenly rises, the kidneys excrete sodium and excess water, causing blood pressure to fall toward normal.

Kidney response to an acute blood pressure rise occurs within several hours and may last for several days. But if high blood pressure continues indefinitely, as in primary hypertension, the kidneys become damaged and begin to lose their ability to deal with the problem.

In addition to regulating blood volume, the kidneys secrete renin and play a crucial role in the neuroendocrine response. We'll discuss the neuroendocrine response in detail beginning on page 12.

**Peripheral resistance.** This force is created by friction between moving blood and peripheral vessel walls—specifically, arteriole walls. The amount of friction depends on both the blood's viscosity and the size of the vessels. A decrease in vessel diameter (for example, from vasoconstriction or arteriosclerosis) increases peripheral resistance and limits blood flow from the arteries into the arterioles. Because this increases arterial blood volume, arterial blood pressure rises. Conversely, vasodilation reduces peripheral resistance and blood pressure drops.

**Understanding autoregulation.** An artery's diameter may change in response to direct nervous stimulation and the influence of neurotransmitter hormones, such as epinephrine, norepinephrine, and angiotensin. (These controls are sometimes called extrinsic mechanisms, because they're initiated outside the circulatory system.) But the artery's diameter also responds directly to local tissue needs through a system of local (or intrinsic) mechanisms. Called *autoregulation*, this system maintains tissue perfusion regardless of systemic blood pressure fluctuations.

The most influential intrinsic mechanisms are *stress relaxation* and *capillary fluid shift*. Stress relaxation enables blood vessels to gradually dilate when blood pressure rises, reducing peripheral resistance and allowing more blood to pass at lower pressure. Capillary fluid shift moves plasma between the vessels and the extravascular compartments. This mechanism, which takes effect more slowly than stress relaxation, helps compensate for a severe rise in pressure (for example, following excessive intravenous fluid infusion) or a severe pressure drop (for example, following massive hemorrhage).

## HOW BLOOD FLOWS: THE BLOOD PRESSURE GRADIENT

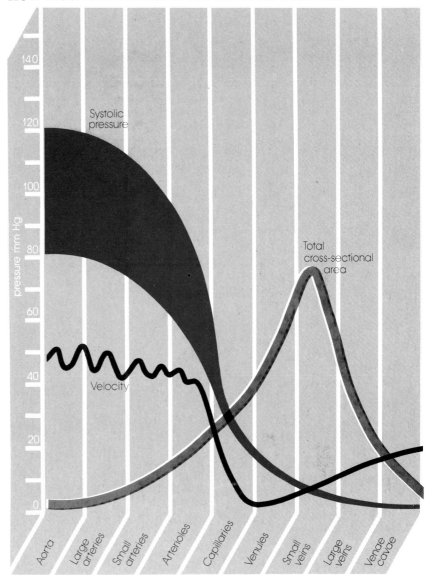

Like all fluid, blood flows from high pressure areas to low pressure areas. In the circulatory system, pressure changes (called the pressure gradient) keep blood flowing from the high-pressure aorta to the low-pressure venae cavae.

This graph illustrates blood flow and velocity throughout the circulatory system. Note that blood velocity drops as the concentration of blood vessels in any given area (total cross-sectional area) increases.

# NEUROENDOCRINE REGULATION

### HOW THE NEUROENDOCRINE SYSTEM RESPONDS TO BLOOD PRESSURE CHANGES

A complex, highly coordinated process of central nervous system and endocrine responses, called the neuroendocrine response, helps keep blood pressure stable. Before you can understand how a disruption in this finely tuned mechanism contributes to hypertension, you have to understand how the neuroendocrine response works. Here's an overview.

**Sensing blood pressure changes.** Blood pressure fluctuates almost continually. The baroreceptors (tension-sensitive sensory receptors) located in the carotid sinus and aortic arch sense these changes and trigger chain reactions designed to maintain blood pressure within safe limits.

To begin tracing the reactions that result, examine the flow-

chart below. Imagine, for instance, that blood pressure decreases slightly. The baroreceptors sense the decrease and send fewer inhibitory impulses to the hypothalamus. Because of this, the hypothalamus is released from inhibition and can send more impulses to the pituitary gland. (Normally, the hypothalamus is inhibited by the

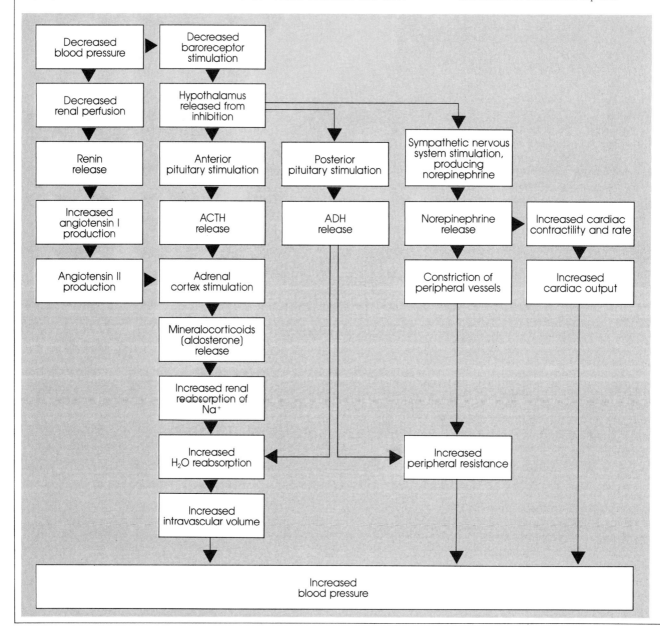

impulses it receives.)

**Pituitary response.** The hypothalamus synthesizes antidiuretic hormone (ADH) and stores it in the *posterior pituitary*. When appropriate, the hypothalamus directs the posterior pituitary to release ADH, which helps conserve blood volume by decreasing water excretion by the kidneys. ADH may also constrict arterioles, which increases peripheral resistance and raises blood pressure.

When stimulated by the hypothalamus, the *anterior pituitary* releases adrenocorticotropic hormone (ACTH), which stimulates the adrenal cortex to release mineralocorticoids (including aldosterone). As shown at left, aldosterone acts on renal tubules to promote reabsorption of sodium and water and the excretion of potassium, which help conserve intravascular fluid.

Because of aldosterone's powerful effects, an excess may result in fluid retention—which, in turn, increases intravascular volume and contributes to high blood pressure. Some diuretics specifically block aldosterone's effects on the kidneys.

**The kidneys' role.** The kidneys play a direct role in the neuroendocrine response by triggering the *renin-angiotensin-aldosterone system*. This important regulatory process begins with a decrease in blood pressure in the arterioles supplying the renal glomeruli (or by a low level of urinary sodium reaching the juxtaglomerular apparatus). This stimulates renin release by the kidneys. Renin acts on one of the blood's plasma proteins (renin substrate) to release angiotensin I. After a complex transformation takes place, angiotensin I is converted into angiotensin II. A potent vasoconstrictor, angiotensin

II also stimulates further secretion of aldosterone by the adrenal cortex, which, as we've already seen, will eventually lead to increased blood pressure.

---

*Keep in mind that the body's capacity to adapt to abnormal conditions, such as repeated or prolonged hypertension, is limited.*

---

**Catecholamine hormones.** Epinephrine and norepinephrine, two catecholamine hormones, are released by the adrenal medulla, in response to sympathetic stimulation. Norepinephrine is also released directly by sympathetic nerve endings. These hormones affect blood pressure as follows:

• *Epinephrine* stimulates the anterior pituitary gland to secrete ACTH; this hormone, in turn, stimulates the adrenal cortex to release mineralocorticoids and glucocorticoids.

Epinephrine also constricts kidney vessels, which stimulates the renin-angiotensin-aldosterone system.

• *Norepinephrine* is primarily a vasoconstrictor. As shown on the previous page, it constricts peripheral vessels, which increases peripheral resistance. In addition, it constricts arteries, thereby helping to raise arterial blood pressure. Norepinephrine also increases cardiac contractility and rate, and constricts kidney vessels.

**Feedback mechanisms.** The neuroendocrine system's built-in safeguards prevent all these mechanisms from raising blood pressure too high. When blood pressure gets too high, feedback mechanisms prevent further release of catecholamines, which, in turn, prevents further vasoconstriction.

Similarly, feedback mechanisms inhibit renin production, slowing the renin-angiotensin-aldosterone system and encouraging a decline in peripheral resistance.

---

### PROSTAGLANDINS: ANOTHER REGULATOR

Prostaglandins, a group of at least 15 hormones derived from fatty acids, are secreted by tissue cells throughout the body. Although many of their functions are not completely understood, researchers believe one type, prostaglandin $E_2$ (PGE$_2$), regulates blood flow through the kidneys by stimulating renal vasodilation, urinary sodium excretion, and renin release. Research indicates that a PGE$_2$ deficiency may cause, or contribute to, primary hypertension.

No one knows exactly what role PGE$_2$ plays in primary hypertension. According to one theory, circulating angiotensin II (produced by the renin-angiotensin-aldosterone system) stimulates the renal medulla to release PGE$_2$. Possibly this hormone antagonizes angiotensin II, which is a potent vasoconstrictor. Thus, PGE$_2$ (along with other vasodilators, such as bradykinin) normally functions as a safeguard against excessive vasoconstriction.

# HYPERTENSION BASICS

## A GLOSSARY OF TERMS

You've heard hypertension described in a variety of ways: acute or chronic (referring to blood vessel changes), benign or malignant (referring to the disease's course), and primary or secondary (referring to the disease's etiology). To be sure you understand these and other related terms, review this glossary.

**Acute hypertension.** A fluid pressure imbalance between intravascular and interstitial fluid, which increases the arterial lining's permeability and permits fluid to shift. Edema and inflammation result.

**Benign hypertension.** Gradual rise in blood pressure with minimal clinical signs. The disease progresses slowly over many years, rarely causing complications until it's far advanced.

**Chronic hypertension.** Thickening of the artery's medial layer from cell proliferation. Lumen narrowing restricts blood flow and reduces elasticity.

**Hypertension.** Sustained high blood pressure (blood pressure readings at levels associated with greater than 50% increase over expected mortality). For details on commonly accepted parameters, see the box below.

**Hypertensive crisis.** Acute, severe, life-threatening blood pressure rise causing rapid deterioration of brain, heart, and kidney function.

**Labile hypertension.** Intermittent high blood pressure.

**Malignant hypertension (accelerated or necrotizing hypertension).** Sudden, sustained rise in blood pressure with dramatic clinical signs. Complications appear early in the disease's course. Fibrinoid necrosis develops in the heart, kidneys, or brain. If untreated, the disease is fatal in about 2 years.

**Primary hypertension (essential or idiopathic hypertension).** Sustained high blood pressure of unknown cause.

**Secondary hypertension.** Sustained high blood pressure caused by an identifiable disease, condition, or drug; for example, pheochromocytoma, renal artery stenosis, or oral contraceptives.

## PRIMARY HYPERTENSION: STILL A MYSTERY

In nursing, few conditions are as puzzling or as frustrating as a disease with no known cause. Primary (idiopathic or essential) hypertension is a perfect example. Although you can explain to your patient why the disease is dangerous and how it may eventually affect his body, you *can't* explain why it developed in the first place.

But you can tell him that certain factors undoubtedly contributed to the disease's development. Although no one understands precisely why, your patient's condition was probably precipitated or aggravated by one or more of the following:

• Diet. Excessive sodium intake, a characteristic of the American diet, leads to water retention, expanded plasma volume, and increased peripheral resistance. All contribute to high blood pressure.

• Stress. Physical as well as emotional stress triggers the neuroendocrine response. This complex set of neurologic and endocrine reactions may cause prolonged vasoconstriction and other components of the fight-or-flight response. Stress also stimulates cholesterol production, which contributes to atherosclerosis.

• Heredity. According to one estimate, a hereditary predisposition to hypertension increases a person's chances of developing it by 30% to 60%. This factor may explain why some people develop hypertension in response to certain stressors, while others successfully adapt.

## RECOGNIZING HYPERTENSION: SOME GUIDELINES

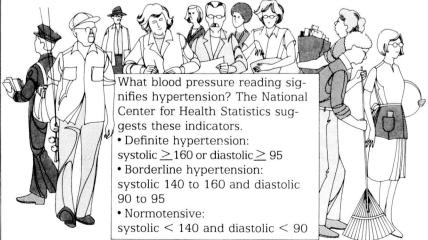

What blood pressure reading signifies hypertension? The National Center for Health Statistics suggests these indicators.
• Definite hypertension: systolic $\geq$ 160 or diastolic $\geq$ 95
• Borderline hypertension: systolic 140 to 160 and diastolic 90 to 95
• Normotensive: systolic < 140 and diastolic < 90

## UNDERSTANDING HYPERTENSION'S EFFECTS

Just as the etiology of primary hypertension is uncertain, the regulatory system disruptions contributing to its progress aren't fully understood. However, the pathologic effects discussed below seem to typify primary hypertension.

**Blood volume.** Excessive sodium retention is a common denominator of primary hypertension. Sodium retention, of course, leads to water retention and expanded blood volume.

Why does your hypertensive patient retain sodium and water? Consider this theory.

Possibly because of a neurogenic excitatory influence, the sympathetic nervous system may be stimulated to release excessive catecholamines. They, in turn, may stimulate the adrenergic receptors in the juxtaglomerular apparatus to release renin. This triggers the renin-angiotensin-aldosterone system.

As you learned on pages 12 and 13, aldosterone influences fluid volume through the control of sodium excretion. If the renin-angiotensin-aldosterone system isn't checked by normal feedback mechanisms, excessive aldosterone production leads to water retention. (For more details on renin's role, see page 16.)

**Peripheral resistance.** In addition to influencing blood volume, the renin-angiotensin-aldosterone system's overstimulation contributes to vasoconstriction, causing increased peripheral resistance. Circulating angiotensin II, a product of the renin-angiotensin-aldosterone system, is a powerful pressor agent that stimulates the receptor sites of smooth muscle and causes vasoconstriction.

As already mentioned, the neurogenic excitatory influence stimulates catecholamine release. One of the most potent catechol-

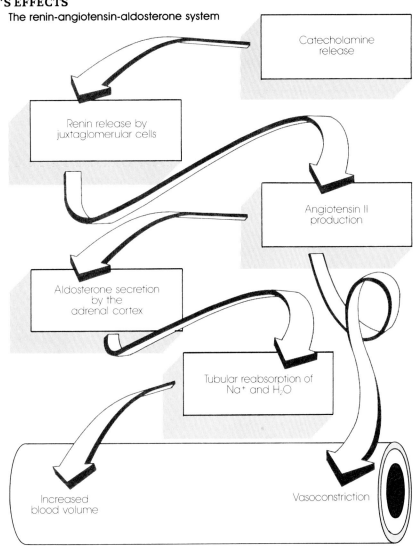

**The renin-angiotensin-aldosterone system**

In primary hypertension, the renin-angiotensin-aldosterone system, which can be stimulated by catecholamine release (as shown here), may help perpetuate hypertension.

amines, norepinephrine, is a powerful vasoconstrictor that increases peripheral vascular resistance.

A deficiency of natural vasodilators may also contribute to high peripheral resistance. Normally, a balance between naturally occurring alpha-adrenergic antagonists (vasodilators) and alpha-adrenergic agonists (vasoconstrictors) helps maintain blood pressure at a stable, safe level. Prostaglandin $E_2$, for instance, normally opposes vasoconstriction in the kidneys. A lack of this substance may precipitate hypertension. Similarly, bradykinin, a peptide found in tissue and plasma, is a vasodilator that normally acts as an adrenergic antagonist. A deficiency of bradykinin may lead to excessive vasoconstriction and hypertension.

# HYPERTENSION BASICS

## RENIN'S ROLE

Because it's indispensable to the renin-angiotensin-aldosterone system, renin indirectly contributes to the increased blood volume and peripheral resistance typical of primary hypertension. Ironically, however, circulating renin levels have no value in your assessment of primary hypertension. As the graph at right shows, renin levels vary widely among patients with primary hypertension, making renin levels unreliable as assessment indicators.

Why such variance? Possibly because renin's effects depend more on the patient's sensitivity to renin than on the amount of renin in the bloodstream.

*Note:* Renin level measurements may be valuable for assessing some types of *secondary* hypertension. For example, high renin levels suggest renovascular hypertension; low renin levels suggest primary aldosteronism.

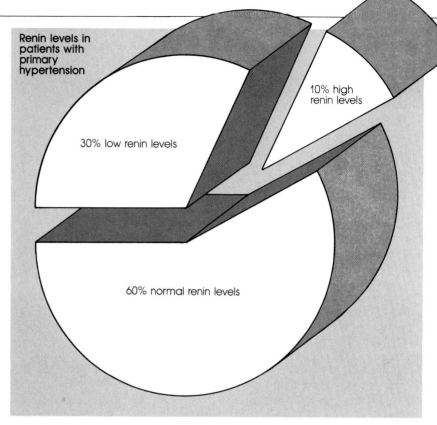

Renin levels in patients with primary hypertension

30% low renin levels

10% high renin levels

60% normal renin levels

## HOW HYPERTENSION AFFECTS BLOOD VESSELS

As hypertension disrupts regulatory mechanisms, those mechanisms actually begin perpetuating hypertension. Eventually, sustained high blood pressure causes pathologic changes in the blood vessels. Let's take a look at the effects of high systolic and diastolic pressures.

**High systolic pressure.** Sustained high systolic blood pressure causes the aorta to lose its elasticity. Vitally important vessels (including the aorta, coronary arteries, basilar artery of the brain, and peripheral vessels in the limbs) become weakened, sclerosed, and tortuous.

In addition, vessel lumens narrow, diminishing the amount of blood they can deliver to tissues. As damage progresses, these vessels can eventually become

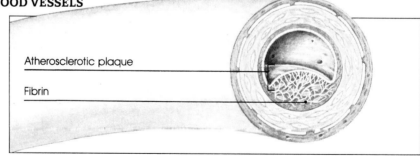

Atherosclerotic plaque

Fibrin

When fibrin accumulates in a blood-vessel's walls (as shown above), the vessel lumen narrows, restricting blood flow through the vessel.

occluded or rupture, causing hemorrhage.

**High diastolic pressure.** Sustained high diastolic pressure causes damage to the small vessels' intima layer. The intima damage causes fibrin, an essential protein required for blood clotting, to accumulate in the vessel walls, possibly occluding the vessels.

As a result of all this vascular damage, blood supply to tissues in the heart, brain, and kidneys drops considerably, eventually causing organ damage (for example, hypertensive heart disease or kidney failure). Read on to find out just how the blood vessel changes can damage certain organs.

## HOW HYPERTENSION AFFECTS ORGANS

The blood vessel deterioration characteristic of primary hypertension eventually damages those organs most dependent on a generous blood supply: the heart, brain, kidneys, and eyes. Here's how uncontrolled hypertension is most likely to affect each of these organs.

**The heart.** To understand why hypertension eventually affects the heart, first consider how the venous system normally protects it from increased blood volume. To protect the heart from overload, veins distend and withhold from 65% to 75% of circulating blood.

In hypertension, increased sympathetic activity, coupled with high peripheral resistance, impairs the venous system's ability to protect the heart from excessive blood volume. Constricted veins lose their ability to distend and store blood, so venous return rises. Now the heart must pump harder and faster to accommodate the added work load.

To compensate, the heart enlarges and increases its contractile force. The left ventricle enlarges to receive the excessive venous return, a process known as *left ventricular dilation.* In addition, the myocardium thickens (a process called *left ventricular hypertrophy*) to increase the contractile strength needed to maintain stroke volume. If the heart fails to compensate for its increased work load, congestive heart failure may result.

Also, coronary arteries fail to supply the hypertrophied left ventricle with enough blood. Sclerotic lesions develop on vessel walls, possibly causing angina pectoris or myocardial infarction.

**The brain.** Inadequate cerebral blood flow, possibly resulting from atherosclerotic lesions, diminishes cerebral perfusion. Decreased perfusion inhibits nerve impulses. Depending on the part of the brain affected, the patient may suffer memory loss, temperament changes, and decreased spontaneity. Eventually his speech, gait, and coordination change. Persistent hypertension may lead to cerebral edema and progressive encephalopathy.

**The kidneys.** Hypertension disturbs kidney circulation by causing fibrinoid necrosis of the afferent arterioles, depriving the glomeruli of oxygen and nutrients. Eventually kidney damage prevents the kidneys from filtering toxic waste, causing uremia and kidney failure.

**The eyes.** In the eyes, hypertension causes vasoconstriction of the arterioles, capillary rupture, and retinopathy (manifested by blurred vision, scotoma, or diminished visual acuity). Optic nerve swelling (papilledema) indicates increased intracranial pressure.

### Heart cross section

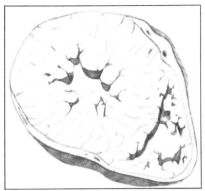

Viewed from the top, this hypertrophied left ventricle contrasts strikingly with the normal-sized right ventricle.

### Intracranial hemorrhage

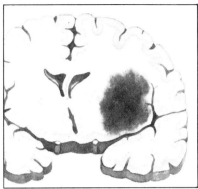

Damage to blood vessels supplying the brain may lead to stroke. In this illustration, note how the hemorrhage has displaced the brain's ventricles.

### Left ventricle: side view

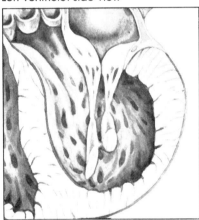

Hypertension may cause the left ventricle to dilate, as shown above.

### Necrotic afferent arteriole

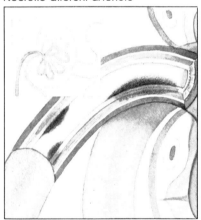

Hypertension may also lead to necrosis in a kidney's afferent arteriole. The inset illustration shows where an afferent arteriole joins a glomerulus.

# SECONDARY HYPERTENSION

## UNDERSTANDING SECONDARY HYPERTENSION

Unlike primary hypertension, secondary hypertension—which accounts for between 5% and 10% of all hypertension cases—has known causes. Many causes of secondary hypertension are curable.

In addition to underlying causes detailed below, these other conditions may lead to secondary hypertension: toxemia of pregnancy, increased intracranial pressure (for example, from a brain tumor or hematoma), and advanced collagen disease. Some drugs (such as oral contraceptives and monoamine oxidase inhibitors) may also trigger hypertension.

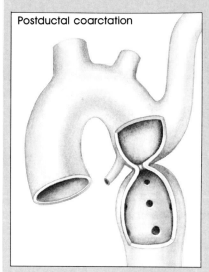

### Postductal coarctation

### COARCTATION OF THE AORTA

Congenital constriction of the aorta, usually just below the left subclavian artery near the site where the ligamentum arteriosum joins the pulmonary artery to the aorta. This condition is classified as *preductal* when it occurs above the ligamentum arteriosum or *postductal* when it occurs below the ligamentum arteriosum.

### Pathophysiology
• Coarctation commonly causes systolic hypertension. Diastolic hypertension also may be present, if coarctation of the abdominal aorta is compromising renal circulation.
• This obstruction of the aorta causes hypertension in the aortic branches above the constriction—the arteries that supply blood to the arms and brain—and diminished blood pressure and pulses in vessels below the constriction. As a result, the patient's legs may be poorly developed.
• Pressure in the left ventricle increases, causing dilation of the proximal aorta and ventricular hypertrophy.
• Collateral circulation above the obstruction may cause the intercostal arteries to dilate, producing rib notching (an important diagnostic sign).
• If a ventricular septal defect accompanies coarctation, blood shunts from left to right, straining the right side of the heart. This leads to pulmonary hypertension and eventually right ventricular hypertrophy and failure.

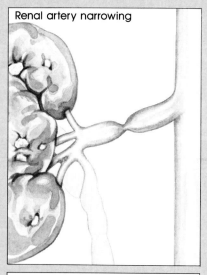

### Renal artery narrowing

### RENOVASCULAR HYPERTENSION

Increased systemic blood pressure, from atherosclerotic narrowing of the renal artery (most common in men age 40 to 70) or fibroplasia of the renal artery's medial layer (most common in women age 20 to 50). Other causes include anomalies of the renal arteries, embolism, tumors and other lesions, dissecting aneurysm, or trauma. This hypertension type affects 1% to 2% of all hypertensive adults.

### Pathophysiology
• Stenosis or occlusion of the renal artery causes ischemia, which stimulates the affected kidney to release excessive amounts of renin and triggers the renin-angiotensin-aldosterone system. Eventually, hypertension damages the unaffected kidney.

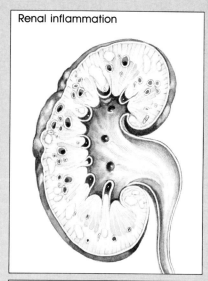

### Renal inflammation

### RENAL PARENCHYMAL DISEASE
### ACUTE AND CHRONIC GLOMERULONEPHRITIS, PYELONEPHRITIS

Immune response to an infection—usually beta hemolytic streptococcal—causing inflammatory changes in the kidneys' interstitia and glomeruli

### Pathophysiology
• Inflammation interferes with the nephrons' excretory ability. Consequently, the kidneys lose their capacity to excrete sodium. Also,

the inflammation interferes with blood flow, triggering the renin-angiotensin-aldosterone system.

• *Pyelonephritis*, a sudden inflammation in the interstitium, may be caused by an infection spreading from the bladder to the ureters, then to the kidneys. Vesicourethral reflux may develop. Chronic pyelonephritis is a persistent kidney infection that leads to kidney scarring and chronic renal failure.

• With *glomerulonephritis*, disease characteristics occur 10 days to 3 weeks after an infection. The kidney becomes swollen, fatty, and congested. A bloody exudate seeps from capillaries, infiltrating renal parenchyma and diminishing renal function.

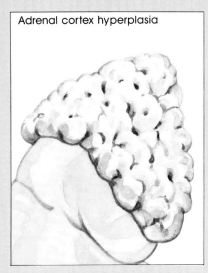

Adrenal cortex hyperplasia

### CUSHING'S SYNDROME

Excessive glucocorticoid secretions by the adrenal cortex

### Pathophysiology

• In about 70% of all cases, excessive amounts of adrenocorticotropic hormone (ACTH) cause hyperplasia of the adrenal cortex. Possible causes are pituitary tumors or tumors in other tissues (sometimes called ectopic ACTH syndrome). An example is bronchogenic oat cell carcinoma.

• In the other 30%, an adrenal tumor secretes cortisol. Cortisol, like aldosterone, promotes sodium reabsorption, and potassium and hydrogen excretion.

• Patients experience persistent hyperglycemia, tissue wasting, and abnormal fat distribution.

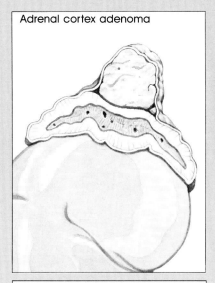

Adrenal cortex adenoma

### HYPERALDOSTERONISM
PRIMARY ALDOSTERONISM OR CONN'S SYNDROME, SECONDARY ALDOSTERONISM, PSEUDOALDOSTERONISM

Excessive aldosterone secretion by the adrenal cortex

### Pathophysiology

• Excessive aldosterone secretion causes excessive sodium reabsorption. As the kidneys reabsorb sodium, they simultaneously excrete potassium and hydrogen. With hyperaldosteronism, increased sodium reabsorption not only increases intravascular fluid volume, but causes an electrolyte imbalance from excessive potassium and hydrogen excretion (resulting in hypokalemia and metabolic alkalosis). Excessive potassium loss may lead to muscle weakness and cardiac arrhythmias.

• *Primary aldosteronism* is caused

by an aldosterone-producing adrenal adenoma in about 75% of all patients; most of these adenomas are benign. Of the remaining patients, most suffer from bilateral adrenal hyperplasia (cell proliferation).

• *Secondary aldosteronism* is usually caused by extra-adrenal pathology that stimulates increased aldosterone production. Ovarian tumors, for example, may secrete aldosterone.

• *Pseudoaldosteronism* is caused by eating large amounts of licorice, which contains glycyrrhizic acid. This chemical is similar to aldosterone in its effects.

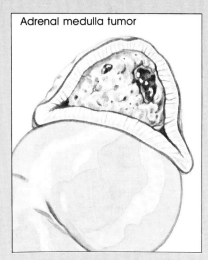

Adrenal medulla tumor

### PHEOCHROMOCYTOMA

Chromaffin tissue tumor, most commonly found in the adrenal medulla. Pheochromocytoma affects only about 0.1% to 0.3% of all hypertensive patients. About 10% of patients with pheochromocytoma have bilateral adrenal pheochromocytoma; about 10% have a malignant tumor.

### Pathophysiology

• The tumor causes excessive secretion of the catecholamines epinephrine and/or norepinephrine. This may cause sustained or paroxysmal hypertension.

# ASSESSING YOUR PATIENT

No one knows what causes primary hypertension. But everyone agrees that early detection is the key to successful management.

In this section, we tell you how to recognize the early stages of hypertension by thoroughly discussing patient assessment. Throughout the discussion, we point out important assessment findings, such as the warning signs of secondary hypertension, and risk factors, such as obesity and diabetes, that should make you suspicious. To help you follow through on your suspicions, we include detailed information on the laboratory tests the doctor may order.

We also review important facts about proper blood pressure measurement. We know you've taken hundreds of blood pressure measurements, but the tips and suggestions we offer will help increase the accuracy of your readings. We'll help you teach your patient and his family about home blood pressure monitoring, too.

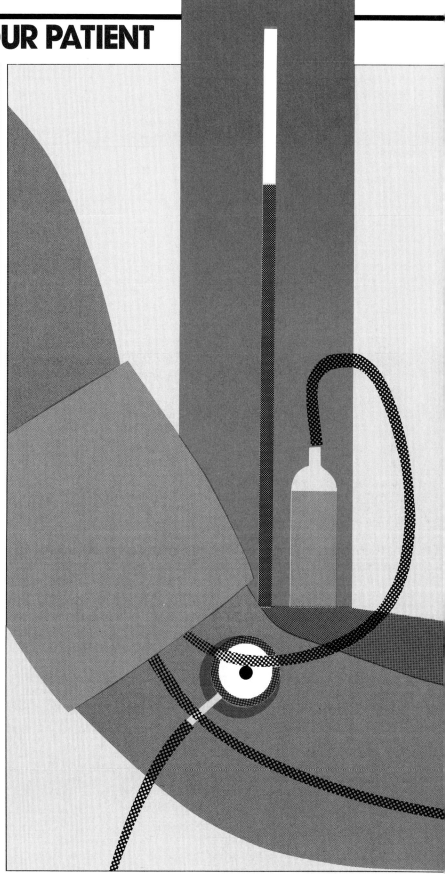

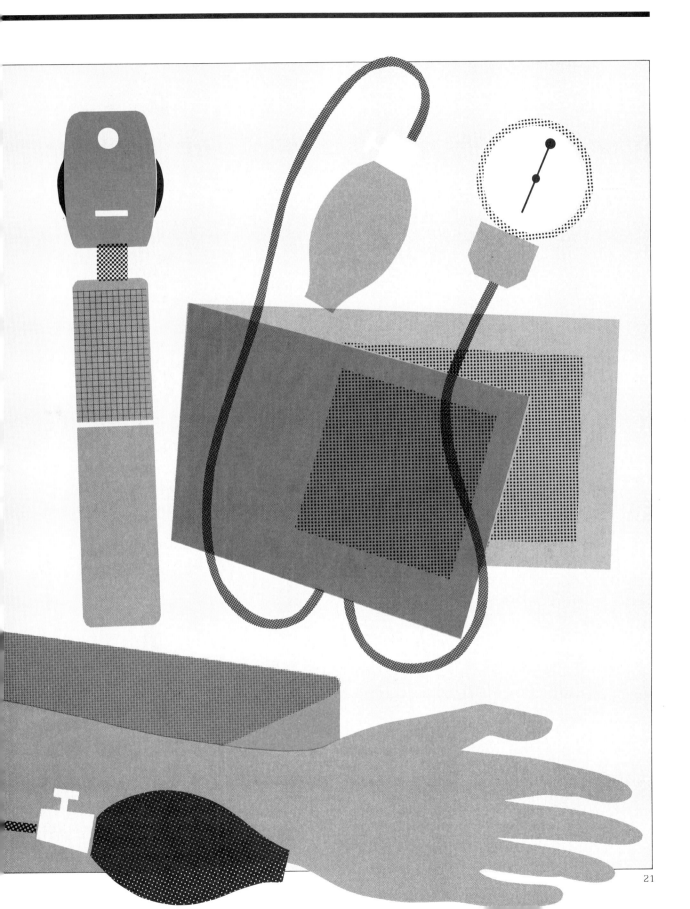

# HEALTH HISTORY

## WHO'S AT RISK?

You've heard hypertension called the silent killer. And no wonder. In its early stages, it works silently, giving no indication of the insidious damage it's doing to blood vessels and vital organs.

In the absence of telltale signs, how can you identify hypertension in its earliest stage? The presence of hypertension risk factors may be your first clue. When you perform an assessment, keep these points in mind.

**Age, race, and sex.** Anyone can develop *primary* or *essential hypertension*—hypertension with no known cause. But statistically, an adult between the ages of 35 and 55 is at particular risk, especially if one or both of his parents had high blood pressure or heart disease. His risk increases significantly if he's black. And hypertensive blacks typically have more severe blood pressure elevations than whites.

Sex is a factor, too. Among people at high risk of hypertension, more men than women actually develop it.

Does a person's risk of developing hypertension increase as he ages? Apparently not. Although systolic blood pressure typically rises slightly after age 50, *diastolic* hypertension rarely develops alone unless it's associated with a pathologic cause.

**Cardiovascular factors.** The risk of developing hypertension and suffering from its complications is further increased by the presence of cardiovascular risk factors. In addition to a family history, risk factors include:
• cigarette smoking
• psychological stress
• sedentary life-style
• diabetes
• hypercholesterolemia.

## SECONDARY HYPERTENSION: DON'T BE MISLED

Tony McNaughton, a 48-year-old tailor, has a family history of heart disease. What's more, he's thin and his blood pressure is now 170/100. For all these reasons, you strongly suspect that he's hypertensive.

But then Mr. McNaughton mentions the headaches, palpitations, and diaphoresis he's been experiencing. And suddenly, you're not so sure about your assessment.

Don't let symptoms like these throw you off the track. Headaches, palpitations, and diaphoresis are important symptoms of pheochromocytoma, one of several causes of *secondary hypertension*—hypertension with a known cause.

For some patients, you'll need to inquire about signs and symptoms of secondary hypertension to complete a thorough health history. Make sure you can recognize telltale clues by reviewing the chart below. *Note:* Other causes of secondary hypertension don't have specific warning signs. They include certain drugs, such as amphetamines, steroids, and oral contraceptives, and excessive licorice intake.

### RECOGNIZING SECONDARY HYPERTENSION

| CAUSES | SIGNS AND SYMPTOMS |
|---|---|
| Hyperaldosteronism | Muscle cramps, weakness, polyuria, hypokalemia |
| Coarctation of the aorta | Headache, lower extremity claudication, leg blood pressure 20 mm Hg less than arm pressure, reduced femoral pulses |
| Renal disease | Dysuria, nocturia, hematuria, recurrent urinary tract infections |
| Flank (renal) trauma | Flank pain and tenderness, fever, vomiting, anorexia, costovertebral tenderness |
| Renal artery stenosis | Recent onset or accelerated hypertensive abdominal bruit on auscultation |
| Cushing's syndrome | Moon face; short, thick neck; prominent abdomen; thin extremities; striae; hirsutism |
| Pheochromocytoma | Sustained hypertension or intermittent hypertension, thinness, headache, sweating, palpitations, elevated fasting blood sugar, orthostatic hypotension, pallor |
| Hyperparathyroidism | Back or skeletal pain (especially when bearing weight) from bone decalcification, lamina dura loss from teeth, hypercalcemia, hypercalciuria, kidney stones and kidney disorders such as nephrocalcinosis, motor dysfunction from neuromuscular depression |

# CRITICAL QUESTIONS

## TAKING A HEALTH HISTORY

The next patient you assess may be hypertensive. Will you be able to detect his condition from his responses during the health history? You will if you ask the right questions about his past and present health status. Of course, you'll specifically question him about hypertension risk factors. But don't forget to investigate other important hypertension indicators, such as cardiovascular risk factors. Make sure you cover all the bases by reviewing the checklist below. *Note:* Before you begin taking a history, help your patient relax as much as possible. Explain how his answers to your questions can help you identify and manage his condition. Then, as you proceed, ask each question slowly and clearly. Encourage complete replies by adopting an open, receptive attitude. Never show negative reactions such as surprise, alarm, distaste, impatience, or annoyance.

• How does your patient describe his present state of health?

• Does he know his usual blood pressure? If so, what is it?

• Has he ever been told he has high blood pressure? If so, who told him? How old was he at the time? What's his highest known blood pressure reading?

• Does he control his blood pressure with diet or medication? If he's on medication, what kind? What are the results so far? Has he experienced any side effects?

• When did he take his last dose?

• Does he ever forget to take his medication? If so, how often? Does he reschedule the missed medication?

• Does he take any other medication; for example, steroids, thyroid hormones, cold capsules or diet pills that contain amphetamines? Remember to document his use of both over-the-counter and prescription drugs.

• Does he modify his diet to keep his blood pressure under control? For example, does he avoid foods that are salty and high in cholesterol and carbohydrates?

• Is he overweight? What's his daily caloric and cholesterol consumption? (Have your patient do a 24-hour recall of all foods he's eaten.)

• Does he consume large amounts of alcohol, licorice, or caffeine?

• Does he smoke? If so, how often? How many packs a day?

• Is he under considerable mental stress?

• What kind of work does your patient do? Does his job require physical exertion?

• Has anyone in his family ever had high blood pressure, heart disease, diabetes, or kidney disease?

• Does he have a history of cardiovascular or cerebrovascular disease?

• Is he diabetic?

• Does he have headaches (especially upon rising in the morning) or experience weakness, paralysis, speech disturbances, or vision disturbances (for example, blurring or vision loss in one eye)?

• Does he complain of orthopnea or nocturnal dyspnea?

• Does he experience dyspnea on exertion, ankle edema, palpitations, fatigue, or anginal-type pain?

• Does he experience intermittent claudication or cold hands and feet?

• Does he have a history of urinary tract infections? Has he complained of dysuria, nocturia, hematuria, or painful urination?

• Does he have a history of renal trauma or gout? Has he ever had an intravenous pyelogram (IVP) or renal arteriogram? If so, what were the results?

• If your patient is female, does she take oral contraceptives or estrogens?

• Does your patient have other signs and symptoms (such as hirsutism or a history of adrenal or parathyroid disease) that may suggest secondary hypertension?

# BLOOD PRESSURE READINGS

## MEANINGFUL BLOOD PRESSURE READINGS: A GUIDE

For any patient, blood pressure measurement is an indispensable assessment indicator. But for a possibly hypertensive patient, this routine assessment procedure takes on added importance.

Because everyone's blood pressure normally fluctuates during the day, no single blood pressure reading is conclusive. For best results, you need to compare your finding with the patient's basal (baseline) blood pressure reading. (See page 25 for details.) But even if you don't know his basal blood pressure, you can make your assessment more meaningful by averaging several consecutive readings. Use the following guidelines:

• Take several blood pressure measurements on the same arm. Between readings, allow the cuff to deflate completely and wait 30 to 60 seconds; otherwise, venous congestion will falsely elevate subsequent diastolic pressure values. Make sure the patient remains in the same position for each reading. Average the results.

• Repeat the procedure on his other arm. *Note:* Blood pressure can vary by as much as 10 mm Hg between arms.

• If practical, follow the same procedure on the thigh. (For guidelines, see page 28.)

• Document your findings.

*Note:* Is your patient taking antihypertensive medication? Take blood pressure readings first while he's lying down, and again while he's standing up. These readings enable you to identify orthostatic blood pressure changes that some antihypertensives may cause.

## EQUIPMENT CHECKUP

Although you may use an aneroid sphygmomanometer more often, the mercury manometer is more accurate. To help compensate for the aneroid sphygmomanometer's shortcomings, follow these guidelines. Calibrate it monthly against a mercury manometer. In addition, routinely check each part of the equipment to ensure that it's in good working condition, using the following chart as a guide. If you identify a defective or inefficient part, replace it or arrange to have it repaired.

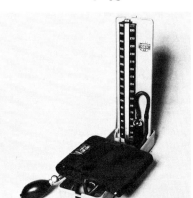

**MERCURY MANOMETER**
**Proper conditions**
• Mercury at zero mark
• Air vent open and clean
**Trouble signs**
• Mercury below or above zero
• Air vent clogged with dirt; signs of oxidation

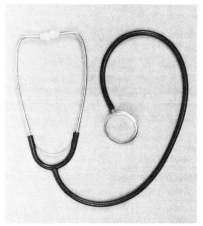

**STETHOSCOPE**
**Proper conditions**
• Tubing soft and pliable, without kinks or tears
• Earpieces clean and snug-fitting
**Trouble signs**
• Dry, cracked tubing (may interfere with sound transmission)
• Dirty, loose-fitting earpieces (may interfere with sound transmission)

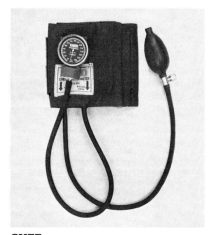

**CUFF**
**Proper conditions**
• Tubing soft and pliable, without kinks or tears
• No tears in cuff fabric
**Trouble signs**
• Hard, dry, cracked tubing (can cause air leaks that may interfere with deflation rate)
• Torn fabric (can cause bulging during inflation, resulting in uneven pressure distribution)

## AVOIDING COMMON PITFALLS

Like most nurses, you've taken hundreds of blood pressure readings. You know the basics inside and out. But even though you're thoroughly familiar with the procedure, you may sometimes overlook the small but important details that ensure the highest degree of accuracy. Avoid common pitfalls by reviewing this checklist.

### Initial steps

• If possible, ask the patient to lie down in a quiet place for about 5 minutes. If he seems tense or anxious, do your best to help him relax.
• Minimize noise and other distractions (for example, from a television or radio).
• Avoid chilly environments, which encourage arteriolar constriction.
• Ask the patient to remove any restrictive clothing, to prevent his blood pressure from becoming artificially elevated.
• Ask him to roll up his sleeve. Never apply the cuff over clothing.
• Comfortably support your patient's arm at heart level, to prevent isometric movement. (Isometric muscle contractions may falsely raise your blood pressure reading.)
• Choose a cuff that's the correct size for your patient. The cuff's bladder width should be about 40% of his arm (or leg) circumference at midpoint; the bladder length should be about 80% of the circumference. A too narrow cuff produces a false-high reading; a too wide cuff produces a false-low reading.

### Performing the procedure

• Apply the blood pressure cuff's bladder directly over your patient's brachial artery, ¾" to 1¼" (2 to 3 cm) above the antecubital space. Center the cuff's bladder over the brachial artery.

• Wrap the cuff snugly. Allow its tubing to hang freely.
• Determine the patient's palpatory systolic blood pressure (see page 26).
• Deflate the cuff and *lightly* apply the stethoscope's diaphragm to the brachial artery. Avoid placing it under the cuff. Make sure the stethoscope tubing hangs freely.

---

*Don't prejudge your patient's blood pressure reading based on his risk factors or previous blood pressure readings. You may unconsciously distort the result.*

---

• Inflate the cuff rapidly and consistently to a pressure 20 to 30 mm Hg above the palpatory systolic pressure. Rapid inflation minimizes the amount of venous blood trapped in the forearm. *Important:* Avoid overinflating the cuff. In addition to causing pain, overinflation may artificially raise blood pressure or cause venospasm.
• Read an aneroid sphygmomanometer's gauge by looking *directly* at it. If you're using a mercury manometer, note the level of the mercury meniscus base when you observe it at eye level.
• Don't make the mistake of deciding your patient has hypertension based on only one blood pressure reading. Look for a hypertensive trend based on at least three readings.
• Document the reading in even numbers.
• Document your patient's position when you took the reading.

## BASAL BLOOD PRESSURE: AN INDISPENSABLE INDICATOR

Everyone's blood pressure varies throughout the day, as a normal function of homeostasis. To accurately assess your patient's blood pressure fluctuations—and identify meaningful variations—you must first establish his baseline (basal) blood pressure.

Basal blood pressure is an average of blood pressure readings taken over 24 hours—ideally, when your patient is relaxed and rested. The doctor may admit the patient to the hospital for basal blood pressure determination, because this setting permits him to control factors that can elevate the patient's blood pressure. These factors include environmental temperature, the patient's emotional stress, diet, cigarette smoking, physical exertion, and conditions such as pain and bladder distention.

To determine your patient's basal blood pressure, take his blood pressure every 3 to 4 hours. At the end of the 24-hour period, average the readings. Document the results.

# BLOOD PRESSURE READINGS

## PROPER CUFF SIZE: MORE IMPORTANT THAN YOU THINK

You know that you should always select a blood pressure cuff that's the appropriate size for your patient's arm. But on a busy day, with many patients to care for, taking the time to fit each patient individually may seem like a low priority. Just how important *is* cuff size, anyway?

According to researchers at the University of California School of Medicine, the wrong cuff size can have a significant effect on your readings. Here's what they discovered.

A cuff that's too small for the patient produces a false-high blood pressure reading. For this reason, 37% of moderately obese patients studied were incorrectly classified as hypertensive, although they actually were normotensive. (Researchers speculate that this factor has caused widespread overestimation of hypertension among obese pa-

tients.) Similarly, a too-large cuff produces a false-low blood pressure reading—leading to the misclassification of some hypertensive patients as normotensive.

Ideally, the researchers suggest that you select an adult cuff size as follows: for arm circumference less than 33 cm, regular; between 33 and 41 cm, large; over 41 cm, thigh-size.

As a practical matter, how can you increase the accuracy of your readings, even if your unit supplies only one cuff size? The chart below provides suggestions for adjusting your readings according to the patient's arm circumference (in centimeters) and the adult cuff size you apply. To use this chart, just add or subtract the number indicated from the diastolic or systolic reading. *Important:* These adjustments aren't standard. Use the proper cuff size whenever possible.

## HOW TO DETERMINE PALPATORY SYSTOLIC PRESSURE

In some patients, Korotkoff sounds temporarily vanish during one of the phases, usually phase II. Called the *auscultatory gap*, this phenomenon may mislead you into recording an erroneously low systolic pressure or, less commonly, an erroneously high diastolic pressure.

Avoid either error by determining your patient's palpatory systolic pressure *before* you take a blood pressure reading. Then, when taking the reading, inflate the cuff 20 to 30 mm Hg higher than this pressure. By doing so, you'll be sure to inflate the cuff adequately for arterial occlusion.

To determine your patient's palpatory systolic pressure, follow this procedure:
• Apply the blood pressure cuff and palpate his radial pulse.
• Rapidly inflate the cuff.
• Note the pressure reading at the point when you no longer feel his radial pulse. Continue to inflate the cuff until the pressure is 20 mm Hg higher than this point.
• Release the air in the cuff at a rate of 2 mm/second. Note the point at which the radial pulse returns. This is the patient's palpatory systolic pressure. As a rule, it's 5 to 10 mm Hg lower than auscultatory systolic pressure. (For details on Korotkoff sounds—including how to augment them when they're hard to hear—see the following page.)

| ARM CIRCUMFERENCE (cm) | CORRECTIONS (mm Hg) | | | | | |
|---|---|---|---|---|---|---|
| | REGULAR CUFF (12 x 23 cm) | | LARGE CUFF (15 x 33 cm) | | THIGH CUFF (18 x 36 cm) | |
| | Systolic | Diastolic | Systolic | Diastolic | Systolic | Diastolic |
| 20 | +11 | +7 | +11 | +7 | +11 | +7 |
| 22 | +9 | +6 | +9 | +6 | +11 | +6 |
| 24 | +7 | +4 | +8 | +5 | +10 | +6 |
| 26 | +5 | +3 | +7 | +5 | +9 | +5 |
| 28 | +3 | +2 | +5 | +4 | +8 | +5 |
| 30 | 0 | 0 | +4 | +3 | +7 | +4 |
| 32 | −2 | −1 | +3 | +2 | +6 | +4 |
| 34 | −4 | −3 | +2 | +1 | +5 | +3 |
| 36 | −6 | −4 | 0 | +1 | +5 | +3 |
| 38 | −8 | −6 | −1 | 0 | +4 | +2 |
| 40 | −10 | −7 | −2 | −1 | +3 | +1 |
| 42 | −12 | −9 | −4 | −2 | +2 | +1 |
| 44 | −14 | −10 | −5 | −3 | +1 | 0 |
| 46 | −16 | −11 | −6 | −3 | 0 | 0 |
| 48 | −18 | −13 | −7 | −4 | −1 | −1 |
| 50 | −21 | −14 | −9 | −5 | −1 | −1 |
| 52 | −23 | −16 | −10 | −6 | −2 | −2 |
| 54 | −25 | −17 | −11 | −7 | −3 | −2 |
| 56 | −27 | −19 | −13 | −7 | −4 | −3 |

**COMPENSATING FOR IMPROPER CUFF SIZE**

Courtesy of *The Lancet*

## REVIEWING KOROTKOFF SOUNDS

Korotkoff sounds are produced by blood movement and vessel vibration as you deflate a blood pressure cuff. As indicated below, these sounds have five phases.

Of course, you'll note systolic pressure when you hear Korotkoff phase I. But not everyone agrees on which Korotkoff phase indicates *diastolic* pressure. Some authorities specify phase IV; others, phase V. As a result, some hospitals require documentation of both phases in addition to phase I; for example, 126/70/66. Check your hospital policy.

**Phase I:** Onset of a faint, clear tapping sound that gradually intensifies.

**Phase II:** Murmur or swishing sound.

**Phase III:** Crisper, louder sounds; more intense tapping sounds.

**Phase IV:** Muffled tapping; softer sound that disappears.

**Phase V:** Silence.

## DEALING WITH THE ABSENT FIFTH PHASE

At some point, you'll take a patient's blood pressure and find that you can't detect phase V of the Korotkoff sounds. In other words, Korotkoff sounds don't disappear, but continue throughout auscultation, until pressure in the cuff is zero.

The absence of this phase prevents you from determining actual diastolic pressure. To correct the problem, first ask yourself the following questions about your blood pressure equipment and your technique:
• Is the blood pressure cuff too small? If it is, the patient's artery probably hasn't been occluded and blood has continued to circulate during the measurement.
• Did you mistakenly place the stethoscope under the cuff?
• Did you apply too much pressure with the stethoscope?

If you discover an error in technique, correct it and try again. Also, try augmenting the Korotkoff signs, using one of the techniques described below. If phase V is still absent despite all your efforts, consider these possible reasons:
• aortic regurgitation
• thyroid toxicosis
• severe anemia
• vigorous exercise shortly before the measurement.

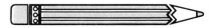

SPECIAL NOTE: If you can't detect the fifth phase, record the pressures at which you hear phase I, phase IV, and the pressure at which you hear the last sound. For example, a blood pressure reading for a patient with an absent fifth phase might look like this: 164/94/0 mm Hg.

## HOW TO AUGMENT KOROTKOFF SOUNDS

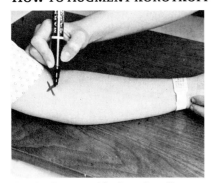

**1** Having trouble hearing Korotkoff sounds? Try to intensify them by increasing vascular pressure below the pressure cuff. Use one of these techniques:

Palpate the brachial pulse and mark it with an indelible marker, as shown above.

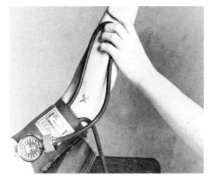

**2** Apply the blood pressure cuff and ask the patient to raise her arm above her head. Support her arm, as shown. Then, rapidly inflate the cuff to a pressure that's 30 mm Hg above her palpatory systolic pressure. Lower her arm so the cuff is at heart level, deflate the cuff, and take a reading.

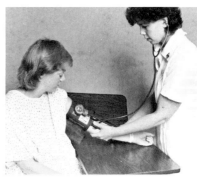

**3** Or, with your patient's arm positioned so the cuff is at heart level, inflate the cuff to 30 mm Hg above her palpatory systolic pressure and ask her to make a fist. Then, have her rapidly open and close her hand about 10 times before you begin to deflate the cuff. Take a reading. CONTINUED ON PAGE 28

## HOW TO AUGMENT KOROTKOFF SOUNDS CONTINUED

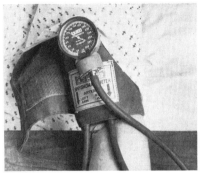

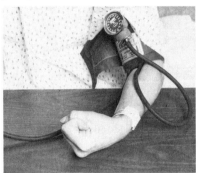

**4** If you're still having difficulty hearing Korotkoff sounds, combine these two techniques. Ask your patient to raise her arm above her head. Rapidly inflate the cuff and have her lower her arm to heart level, as shown here.

**5** Then, have her clench and unclench her fist several times before taking a reading.

Whenever you use one of these techniques, document your reading with the symbol Ka (Korotkoff augmented); for example, 180/100(Ka). This way, the next nurse who takes your patient's blood pressure knows that her Korotkoff sounds are hard to hear and need augmenting.

### SOLVING SPECIAL PROBLEMS

Consider these situations:
• Jack McCabe suffered traumatic injuries in a car accident. Because both his arms are broken, you can't use them for blood pressure measurements.
• Mildred Connors is obese. Because her upper arms are so large, none of your blood pressure cuffs fits properly.

How can you cope with these two special problems? For Mr. McCabe, measuring blood pressure in the thigh may be the answer. For Ms. Connors, consider taking a forearm measurement. For guidelines, read on.

**Measuring blood pressure in the thigh.** Select a cuff that's wide enough and long enough to accommodate the larger circumference of the patient's thigh. (Review the guidelines on pages 25 and 26.) Have the patient lie prone and apply the cuff's bladder over the posterior aspect of his mid-thigh. Place your stethoscope over the popliteal artery in the popliteal fossa. Listen for Korotkoff sounds as in a standard arm measurement.

If your patient can't lie prone, position him supine and flex his leg at the knee. Put your stethoscope over the popliteal fossa. (Expect systolic pressure in the thigh to be 10 to 40 mm Hg higher than in an arm. Diastolic pressure is usually the same.)

**Measuring blood pressure in the forearm.** Select a cuff that's appropriate for the circumference of your patient's forearm. Position it about 5″ (13 cm) from the elbow and proceed as for upper arm measurement. Listen for Korotkoff sounds over the radial artery at the wrist.

## VITAL ORGAN DAMAGE: WHAT YOU SHOULD KNOW

Has hypertension damaged your patient's brain, heart, and kidneys? That depends on how high his blood pressure is, how long it's been elevated, and how well his vessels have accommodated the increased pressure.

High blood pressure doesn't necessarily damage all vital organs. But when damage occurs, it can lead to such devastating complications as stroke, heart failure, and kidney failure. That's why, during your physical assessment, you need to watch for the early signs of damage or dysfunction in these major organs. The following pages provide guidelines.

### MORTALITY RATES

To better understand the impact of vital organ damage, review these results of a mortality study recently reported by the Hypertension Detection and Follow-up Program. They detail the causes of death in a five-year period for 768 hypertensive patients between ages 30 and 69. (These figures exclude violent deaths.)

| | |
|---|---:|
| Cardiovascular diseases | 60.7% |
|   cerebrovascular disease | 11.3% |
|   myocardial infarction | 16.8% |
|   other ischemic heart diseases | 22.1% |
|   hypertensive heart disease | 1.7% |
|   other hypertensive diseases | 1.5% |
|   other cardiovascular diseases | 7.3% |
| Non-cardiovascular diseases | 39.3% |
|   renal disease | 3.5% |
|   diabetes mellitus | 2.1% |
|   other | 33.7% |

## ASSESSING FOR VITAL ORGAN DAMAGE

To assess your patient for possible vital organ damage, take a systematic, head-to-toe approach as indicated in the following chart. Thoroughly document your findings.

| | PROCEDURE | ABNORMAL FINDINGS | POSSIBLE IMPLICATIONS |
|---|---|---|---|
| **NECK** | • Auscultate the carotid arteries. | • Bruits | • Atherosclerosis<br>• Stenosis<br>• Occlusion |
| | • Inspect the neck. | • Distended jugular veins | • Elevated central venous pressure<br>• Right heart failure |
| | • Palpate the thyroid gland. | • Enlarged thyroid gland | • Hyperparathyroidism (a possible cause of secondary hypertension) |
| **CHEST** | • Palpate the point of maximal impulse (PMI) located at the left fifth intercostal space, just medial to the midclavicular line. | • Lateral displacement | • Left ventricular hypertrophy |
| | • Turn the patient on his left side and listen with the stethoscope's bell for heart sounds. | • $S_4$, or atrial gallop. (One of the first auscultatory changes in hypertension. An $S_4$ is present in most hypertensive patients.) | • Rigid left ventricle |
| | | • $S_3$, or ventricular gallop. (In children and young adults, $S_3$ is normal.) | • Early congestive heart failure |
| | • Place the stethoscope's diaphragm over the second intercostal space at the right sternal border. | • Accentuated $S_2$ | • Hypertension |
| | • Auscultate the lungs. | • Rales, wheezing | • Congestive heart failure |
| **ABDOMEN** | • Inspect the abdomen. | • Abundance of pink-purplish striae | • Cushing's syndrome (a possible cause of secondary hypertension) |
| | • Palpate the abdominal quadrants for softness, firmness, tenderness, and masses. (For information on kidney palpation, see the photostory on pages 30 to 31.) | • Masses, tenderness | • Renal disease (renal artery stenosis) |
| | • Use the stethoscope's bell to auscultate the abdomen. | • Bruits | • Renal disease |
| **LEGS** | • Inspect the feet and legs for skin color, lesions, edema, hair distribution, and temperature. | • Edema<br>• Skin discoloration, hair loss, coldness | • Heart failure<br>• Peripheral vascular disease |
| | • Palpate the peripheral pulses (femoral, popliteal, posterior tibial, dorsalis pedis) for rate, quality, and equality. | • Diminished or delayed femoral pulse<br>• Diminished, delayed, or absent pulses | • Coarctation of the aorta<br>• Occlusive aortic disease |
| | • Auscultate the femoral artery. | • Bruits | • Turbulent blood flow from atherosclerosis or aneurysm |

# VITAL ORGANS

## HOW TO PALPATE YOUR PATIENT'S KIDNEYS

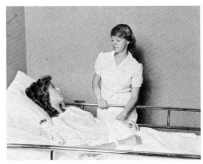

**1** Begin by explaining the procedure to your patient and answering her questions.
   *Caution:* If you suspect pheochromocytoma, don't palpate the kidney. Palpation may cause an acute hypertensive episode.

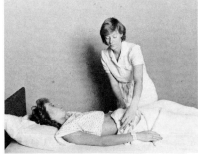

**2** Then, place her in a supine position. Expose her abdomen from her xiphoid process to her symphysis pubis. Warm your hands before proceeding further.

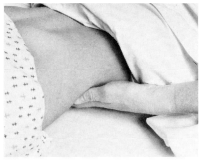

**3** Stand by her right side and place your left hand underneath her, as shown here—midway between the lower costal margin and iliac crest.

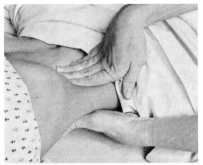

**6** Normally, kidneys are difficult to palpate. If you can't feel your patient's kidneys, try using another palpation technique called *capturing the kidney*. Begin with the right kidney, as shown here. Position your hands as you did in Step 4. Then, ask your patient to inhale deeply. At the peak of her inhalation, quickly but gently press your hands together.

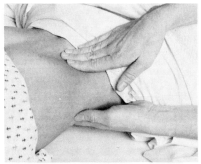

**7** Now ask your patient to exhale slowly. When she's finished, slowly release your hands. You may feel the kidney slide between your hands. If the kidney's palpable, note its contour and check for lumps, masses, or tenderness. Mentally note the kidney's size.

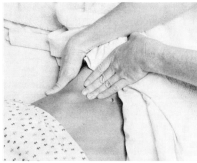

**8** Then, using the same method, attempt to palpate her left kidney. (It's usually located slightly higher than the right kidney.) If you're able to do so, compare its size and contour to the right kidney's. If one kidney is smaller than the other, it may be malfunctioning.

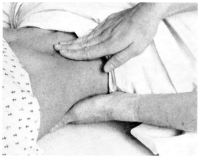

**4** Position your right hand on her abdomen, directly above your left hand. Angle your right hand slightly toward the costal margin, as the nurse is doing here.

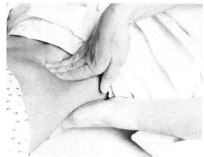

**5** Now, lift up with your left hand as you press down with your right. Each time your patient inhales, press your right hand deeper into her abdomen, until you reach the maximum palpation depth. Ask her to inhale deeply. Expect to feel the lower pole of her right kidney move down between your hands. Note the kidney's contour and size, and check for lumps, masses, or tenderness. Palpate the left kidney.

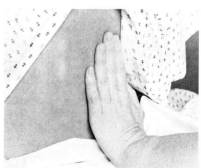

**9** To complete your physical assessment of the patient's kidneys, ask her to sit up. Place your left palm on her back, slightly to the right of her costovertebral angle.

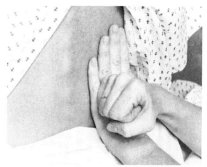

**10** Hit the back of your left hand with your right fist. If your patient feels pain, she may have a kidney infection. Repeat the procedure on her left side.

Document all your assessment findings.

## BRAIN INVOLVEMENT: LOOKING FOR CLUES

Assessing your patient for possible brain involvement isn't easy. Most clues come from careful questioning of the patient and his family, and your own observations. As part of your assessment, look for evidence of neurologic changes, such as speech impairment, decreased coordination, and numbness or weakness in one or more of his extremities. Even subtle indications of neurologic changes, such as slightly slurred speech, can be significant. Also, ask your patient if he's experienced any temporary vision loss or blurring, dizziness, weakness or numbness, or difficulty swallowing. Finally, ask a family member or friend if the patient's personality or behavior has changed recently, if he's become less spontaneous, and if he's become forgetful. Document any signs and symptoms that suggest the possibility of brain infarction, hemorrhage, or other neurologic involvement.

# RETINAL ASSESSMENT

Rheostat

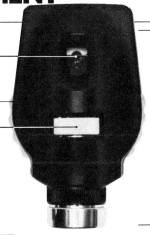

Lens selection dial

Aperture selection dial

Ophthalmoscope head

Handle

## RECOGNIZING HYPERTENSIVE RETINOPATHY

As the next part of your physical assessment, examine your patient's retinas with an ophthalmoscope. Whether his hypertension is acute or mild, you may not observe any abnormalities. Visible changes are especially unlikely if your patient's arteries are still young and resilient and have withstood high blood pressure for only a short time.

But if your patient's hypertension is chronic and severe, you'll probably observe a number of retinal changes during your ophthalmoscopic examination. Known as hypertensive retinopathy, these changes include:
• sclerosis
• constriction of the arterioles and retinal arteries
• hemorrhages
• exudates
• papilledema.

With the exception of sclerosis, these hypertension-related retinal changes, although acute, are usually reversible.

As hypertensive retinopathy progresses, your patient will experience vision changes resulting from retinal deterioration. These changes include blurred vision, scotoma, and loss of visual acuity. Take care to question him about vision changes he's noticed and to test his visual acuity. Document your findings and his responses.

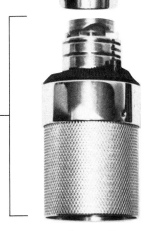

## ASSEMBLING AN OPHTHALMOSCOPE

To properly examine your patient's retinas, you must be skillful at using an ophthalmoscope like the Welch Allyn instrument shown here. Although nothing takes the place of practice, the information and photos on the following pages review the basics.

To assemble this ophthalmoscope, follow these steps:
• Screw the handle onto the battery housing.
• Align the slots in the base of the ophthalmoscope head with the lugs on the handle.
• Firmly push down the head and rotate it clockwise until it clicks into place.

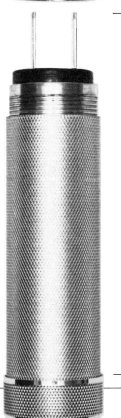

Battery housing

## FOCUSING ON THE RETINA

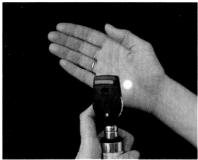

**1** After assembling your ophthalmoscope, turn on its light. Holding the ophthalmoscope about 6" (15 cm) away from your hand, rotate the aperture selection dial on the back of the instrument's head, until you see the correct aperture reflected on your hand. For most patients, choose the large, clear aperture. *Note:* You may use a color or grid aperture for a more detailed assessment.

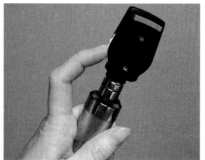

**2** Set the lens selection dial on 0 (neutral). If both you and your patient have normal vision, this setting will probably bring the retina into focus. But to compensate for imperfect vision—yours *or* hers—you may need to readjust the dial when you look into her eye.

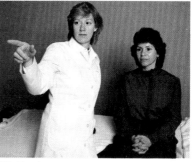

**3** Darken the room to encourage the patient's pupils to dilate. Ask your patient to focus on a stationary object at eye level. This also encourages pupil dilation and helps prevent eye movement.

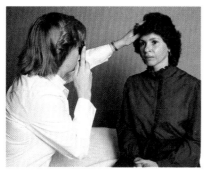

**4** Then, to examine her right eye, hold the ophthalmoscope up to your right eye with your right hand, as shown here. (Do the opposite to examine her left eye.) Steady her head with your hand. Holding the ophthalmoscope at a slight lateral angle about 12" (30 cm) in front of her, direct the light beam into her eye and slowly move the ophthalmoscope closer until you're about 6" from the eye. Look for the red reflex.

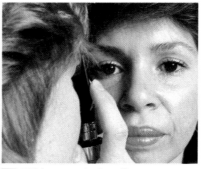

**5** With your index finger on the lens selection dial, slowly move the ophthalmoscope closer to her eye until you see a retinal structure, such as a blood vessel. Focus the ophthalmoscope as necessary by rotating the lens selection dial. Moving your head and the ophthalmoscope as one unit, follow the blood vessel inward until you see the optic disk.

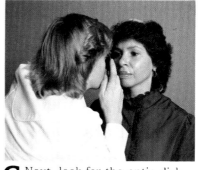

**6** Next, look for the optic disk cup (physiologic cup) at the disk's center or temporal edge. Examine the optic disk and surrounding retina for abnormalities. (To compare a normal retina with several abnormal ones, examine the photos on pages 34 and 35.)

CONTINUED ON PAGE 34

# RETINAL ASSESSMENT

## FOCUSING ON
### THE RETINA CONTINUED

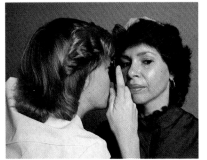

**7** To examine the periphery, ask your patient to first look up, then to the left and the right. To locate the macula, find the disk and look temporally about two disk diameters away. Ask the patient to look directly at the light (or angle the light laterally). Normally, the macula is darker than the retina; the reflective spot at its center is the fovea. *Note:* Because the macula is so sensitive to light, the patient may blink and tear.

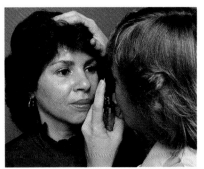

**8** Repeat the entire examination on her left eye. Document all observations (including such abnormalities as an absent red reflex), and note the size and location of lesions according to the guidelines on page 36. Also document the lens selection you used to focus on the retina.

## RECOGNIZING ABNORMALITIES

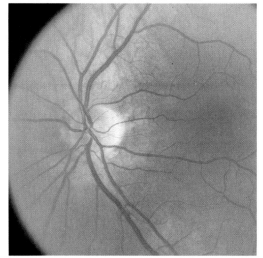

This is a normal fundus. Compare it with the following photos, which depict abnormalities characteristic of hypertension.

As you can see, a normal optic disk is round (or sometimes oval) and yellowish. Its nasal edge is less distinct than the temporal edge. Note that the veins are slightly darker and larger in diameter than the arteries.

◄————

In this photo, you see segmental narrowing of arteries and cotton wool patches—large areas of whitish material that appears fluffy.

————►

In addition to cotton wool patches, the photo at left shows a flame-shaped hemorrhage.

◄————

At right, the fundus is heavily covered with exudates. In contrast to cotton wool patches, exudates are usually yellow and smaller, with more distinct margins.

————►

The silver-colored arteries (called silver wiring) indicate arteriosclerosis. In this photo, the arteries are occluded.

◄————

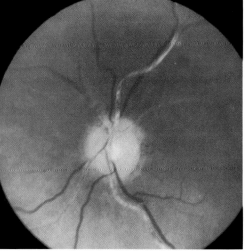

This photo illustrates the ravages of malignant hypertension. Note the arteriovenous nicking and papilledema, which is characterized by swelling of the optic disk and blood vessels.

————►

Photo of retinal abnormalities courtesy of Wills Eye Hospital, Philadelphia

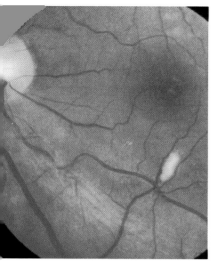

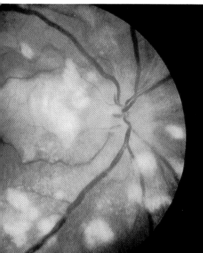

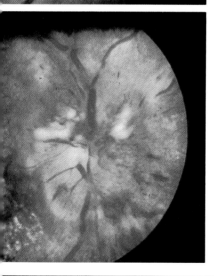

## HYPERTENSIVE RETINOPATHY: DETERMINING ITS SEVERITY

You can determine the severity of your patient's hypertension by observing retinal changes. For guidelines, refer to the Keith-Wagener-Barker scale represented below. As indicated, classify the findings from your ophthalmoscopic examination into one of five grades.

*Note:* The retinal changes caused by hypertension are similar to those caused by arteriosclerosis. To provide effective therapy, the doctor must determine the cause of any abnormalities you observe. Keep in mind, however, that hemorrhages, exudates, and papilledema are abnormalities that *always* call for immediate intervention.

| GRADE | RETINAL CHANGES | IMPLICATIONS |
|---|---|---|
| 0 | • None; eyegrounds (fundus) normal | Normal blood pressure |
| I | • Mild sclerosis | Early or mild hypertension |
| II | • Marked sclerosis<br>• Wide arterial light reflex from thickening and opacity of arterial wall<br>• Veins compressed at arteriovenous crossings<br>• General and focal arterial narrowing (or spasm) | More advanced hypertension |
| III | • Retinal edema<br>• Cotton wool exudates<br>• Hemorrhages (linear or flame-shaped)<br>• Diffuse and focal arterial narrowing (or spasm) | Severe, chronic hypertension |
| IV | • All Grade III signs<br>• Papilledema | Malignant hypertension, including brain involvement |

# RETINAL ASSESSMENT

## DOCUMENTING A LESION'S LOCATION AND SIZE

Suppose you see a retinal hemorrhage, exudate, cotton wool patch, or other lesion. How can you clearly document it? Adopt this method.

First, note the lesion's clockface position. As shown below, a lesion is located at 8:00. Then, using the optic disk's diameter (DD) as a standard, note the lesion's dimensions; for example, ½ DD x ½ DD. Finally, determine the lesion's distance from the disk, again using the disk's diameter as the unit of measurement. Document your findings.

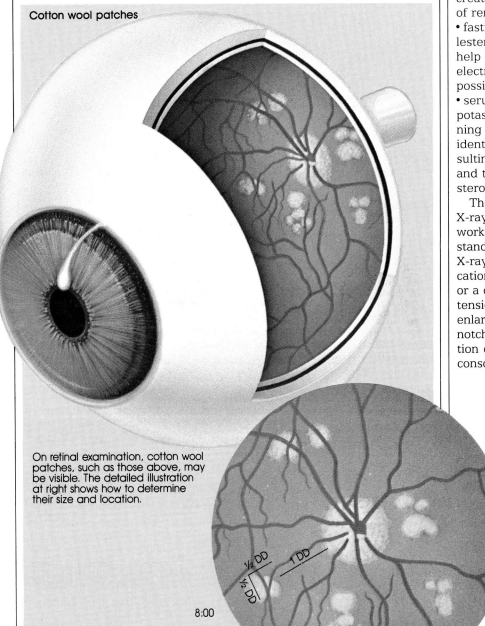

Cotton wool patches

On retinal examination, cotton wool patches, such as those above, may be visible. The detailed illustration at right shows how to determine their size and location.

½ DD    1 DD
½ DD

8:00

# LAB TESTS

## ROUTINE TESTING: WHAT TO EXPECT

To help assess your hypertensive patient, expect the doctor to order these routine tests:
• complete blood cell count
• urinalysis (for evidence of primary renal disease)
• blood urea nitrogen (BUN) and creatinine (to evaluate the extent of renal dysfunction, if present)
• fasting blood sugar, serum cholesterol, uric acid, and EKG (to help evaluate cardiovascular risk, electrophysiologic changes, and possible cardiac damage)
• serum potassium (to evaluate potassium levels before beginning diuretic drug therapy, to identify possible hypokalemia resulting from diuretic therapy, and to screen for primary aldosteronism).

The doctor may include a chest X-ray as part of the patient's workup, although an X-ray isn't standard for all patients. A chest X-ray may reveal either complications of primary hypertension or a cause of secondary hypertension. Possible findings include enlarged heart, dilated aorta, notched ribs (indicating coarctation of the aorta), and patchy consolidations in the lungs.

# SECONDARY HYPERTENSION: LOOKING FOR THE CAUSE

If the doctor suspects that your patient's hypertension has a secondary cause, he'll order specific laboratory tests to confirm his suspicions. In this chart, you'll learn which tests are appropriate, according to the doctor's tentative diagnosis.

Because these additional tests are expensive, the doctor will order them only if the patient is at particular risk of secondary hypertension. Appropriate circumstances include the following:
• Your patient is less than age 20 or more than age 50.
• His hypertension is of rapid onset (especially if he has no family history of hypertension).
• Routine laboratory test results suggest secondary hypertension.
• He doesn't respond to antihypertensive therapy.
• His hypertension suddenly worsens.
• He develops an abdominal bruit.

| RENAL PARENCHYMAL DISEASE: |
| :---: |
| GLOMERULONEPHRITIS, CHRONIC PYELONEPHRITIS, POLYCYSTIC KIDNEYS |

## DIAGNOSTIC TEST

Intravenous pyelogram (IVP)

**Normal findings**
• No soft or hard tissue lesions
• No mucosal abnormalities
• Minimal residual urine
• Prompt visualization of contrast medium in kidneys

**Significant abnormal findings**
• In severe or chronic pyelonephritis, destruction, distortion, and fibrosis of renal tissue with reduced or tortuous vascularity
• With renal abscesses or inflammatory masses, an increase in capsular vessels and abnormal intrarenal circulation

**Interfering factors**
*Poor quality film caused by:*
• Feces or gas in colon
• Injection of insufficient contrast medium
• Recent gastrointestinal or gallbladder series

## DIAGNOSTIC TEST

Renal angiography

**Normal finding**
• Normal appearance of vascular tree and renal parenchyma

**Significant abnormal findings**
• Noticeable constriction in blood vessels
• Presence of renal masses
• Destruction, distortion, and fibrosis of tissue

**Interfering factors**
• A recent barium enema, upper gastrointestinal (GI) series, or other contrast study (may cause cloudy radiogram)
• Feces or gas in GI tract (may cause cloudy radiogram)
• Patient movement during test

| RENOVASCULAR ATHEROSCLEROSIS, RENAL ARTERY STENOSIS |
| :---: |

## DIAGNOSTIC TEST

Rapid sequence IVP

**Normal findings**
• No soft or hard tissue lesions
• No mucosal abnormalities
• Minimal residual urine
• Prompt visualization of contrast medium in kidneys

**Significant abnormal findings**
• In severe or chronic pyelonephritis, destruction, distortion, and fibrosis of renal tissue with reduced or tortuous vascularity

• With renal abscesses or inflammatory masses, an increase in capsular vessels and abnormal intrarenal circulation

**Interfering factors**
*Poor quality film caused by:*
• Feces or gas in colon
• Injection of insufficient contrast medium
• Recent gastrointestinal or gallbladder series

## DIAGNOSTIC TEST

Plasma renin activity (PRA)

**Normal findings**
*Sodium-depleted, upright, peripheral vein:*
• Ages 20 to 39: 2.9 to 24 ng/ml/hr; mean, 10.8 ng/ml/hr
• Ages 40 and over: 2.9 to 10.8 ng/ml/hr; mean, 5.9 ng/ml/hr
*Sodium-replete, upright:*
• Ages 20 to 39: 0.1 to 4.3 ng/ml/hr; mean, 1.9 ng/ml/hr
• Ages 40 and over: 0.1 to 3.0 ng/ml/hr; mean, 1 ng/ml/hr

**Significant abnormal finding**
• Elevated renin levels

**Interfering factors**
• Improper patient positioning during test
• Failure to use proper anticoagulant collection tube, to completely fill tube, or to adequately mix the specimen and the anticoagulant
• Failure to chill the collection tube and syringe, or failure to chill and immediately send the specimen to the laboratory. (Either may promote renin breakdown.)
• These substances and factors may increase plasma renin levels: diuretics, vasodilators, and other antihypertensive drugs; oral contraceptives; licorice; sodium intake; severe blood loss; and pregnancy.

CONTINUED ON PAGE 38

# LAB TESTS

SECONDARY HYPERTENSION: LOOKING FOR THE CAUSE CONTINUED

• These factors may decrease plasma renin levels: salt-retaining steroid therapy and antidiuretic therapy with vasopressin.

### DIAGNOSTIC TEST

Renal vein renin concentration
*Note:* Specimens for this test are taken from both the renal vein and the inferior vena cava; results are then compared.

**Normal finding**
• Renal venous renin ratio (renin level in the renal vein compared with renin level in the inferior vena cava) less than 1.5/1.0

**Significant abnormal finding**
• Elevated renin levels

**Interfering factors**
• Improper patient positioning during test
• Failure to use proper anticoagulant collection tube, to completely fill tube, or to adequately mix the specimen and the anticoagulant
• Failure to chill the collection tube and syringe, or failure to chill and immediately send the specimen to the laboratory. (Either may promote renin breakdown.)
• These substances and factors may increase plasma renin levels: diuretics, vasodilators, and other antihypertensive drugs; oral contraceptives; licorice; sodium intake; severe blood loss; and pregnancy.
• These factors may decrease plasma renin levels: salt-retaining steroid therapy and antidiuretic therapy with vasopressin.

### DIAGNOSTIC TEST

Renal angiogram

**Normal finding**
• Normal appearance of vascular tree and renal parenchyma

**Significant abnormal findings**
• Noticeable constriction in blood vessels
• Presence of renal masses
• Destruction, distortion, and fibrosis of tissue

**Interfering factors**
• A recent barium enema, upper gastrointestinal (GI) series, or other contrast study (may cause cloudy radiogram)
• Feces or gas in GI tract (may cause cloudy radiogram)
• Patient movement during test

## HYPERALDOSTERONISM

### DIAGNOSTIC TEST

Serum aldosterone

**Normal findings**
*Adult in supine position (for at least 2 hours):*
• 7.4 ± 4.2 ng/dl
*Adult in standing position (for at least 2 hours):*
• 13.2 ± 8.9 ng/dl

**Significant abnormal finding**
• Elevated serum aldosterone levels

**Interfering factors**
• Hemolysis from rough handling of specimen
• Patient's failure to observe restrictions of posture and diet
• Antihypertensives, diuretics, and steroids or corticosteroids. (Respectively, these drugs may suppress, raise, and lower aldosterone levels.)
• Recent (within 1 week) radioactive scan

### DIAGNOSTIC TEST

Urine aldosterone

**Normal finding**
• 2 to 16 mcg/24 hr

**Significant abnormal finding**
• Elevated urine aldosterone levels

**Interfering factors**
• Antihypertensive drugs, diuretics, and corticosteroids. (Respectively, these drugs may suppress, raise, and lower aldosterone levels.)
• Patient's failure to maintain normal dietary intake of sodium
• Failure to collect *all* urine during the 24-hour specimen collection period
• Improper specimen storage
• Strenuous physical exercise or emotional stress (may increase aldosterone levels)
• Recent (within 1 week) radioactive scan

### DIAGNOSTIC TEST

Plasma renin activity (PRA)

**Normal findings**
*Sodium-depleted, upright, peripheral vein:*
• Ages 20 to 39: 2.9 to 24 ng/ml/hr; mean, 10.8 ng/ml/hr
• Ages 40 and over: 2.9 to 10.8 ng/ml/hr; mean, 5.9 ng/ml/hr
*Sodium-replete, upright:*
• Ages 20 to 39: 0.1 to 4.3 ng/ml/hr; mean, 1.9 ng/ml/hr
• Ages 40 and over: 0.1 to 3.0 ng/ml/hr; mean, 1 ng/ml/hr

**Significant abnormal finding**
• Decreased renin levels

**Interfering factors**
• Improper patient positioning during test
• Failure to use proper anticoagulant collection tube, to completely fill tube, or to adequately mix the specimen and the anticoagulant

- Failure to chill the collection tube and syringe, or failure to chill and immediately send the specimen to the laboratory. (Either may promote renin breakdown.)
- These factors may increase plasma renin levels: diuretics, vasodilators, and other antihypertensive drugs; oral contraceptives; licorice; sodium intake; severe blood loss; and pregnancy.
- These factors may decrease plasma renin levels: salt-retaining steroid therapy and antidiuretic therapy with vasopressin.

## DIAGNOSTIC TEST

Abdominal computerized tomography (CT)
*Note:* This test may be performed with or without contrast dye.

**Normal finding**
- Renal parenchyma appears slightly more dense than the liver, but less dense than bone.

**Significant abnormal findings**
- Density differences suggesting renal masses
- Confined, usually detached masses, indicating adrenal tumors

**Interfering factors**
- Patient movement during test may blur images.
- Catheters, surgical clips, or recent contrast studies may impair visualization.

## PHEOCHROMOCYTOMA

## DIAGNOSTIC TEST

Vanillylmandelic acid (VMA)

**Normal finding**
- 0.7 to 6.8 mg/24 hr urine collection

**Significant abnormal finding**
- Elevated urine VMA levels

**Interfering factors**
- Methyldopa, theophylline, norepinephrine, epinephrine, ephedrine, lithium carbonate, and methocarbamol (may raise urine VMA levels)
- Chlorpromazine, guanethidine, reserpine, monoamine oxidase (MAO) inhibitors, clonidine (may lower VMA levels)
- Levodopa, salicylates (may raise or lower VMA levels)
- Failure to observe dietary restrictions, if appropriate.
  *Note:* Depending on the laboratory's equipment, dietary restrictions may be unnecessary. Check with your lab for guidelines.
- Failure to collect all urine during the 24-hour period
- Improper specimen storage
- Excessive physical exercise or emotional stress (may raise VMA levels)

## DIAGNOSTIC TESTS

Urine catecholamines
Metanephrines (metanephrines, normetanephrines)

**Normal findings**
*24-hour specimen:*
- Undetectable to 135 mcg
*Random specimen:*
- Undetectable to 18 mcg

**Significant abnormal finding**
- Elevated urine catecholamine

**Interfering factors**
- Caffeine, insulin, nitroglycerin, aminophylline, ethanol, sympathomimetics, methyldopa, tricyclic antidepressants, chloral hydrate, quinidine, quinine, tetracycline, B-complex vitamins, isoproterenol, levodopa, MAO inhibitors (may raise urine catecholamine levels)
- Clonidine, guanethidine, reserpine, iodine-containing contrast media (may suppress urine catecholamine levels)

- Phenothiazines, erythromycin, methenamine compounds (may raise or suppress levels)
- Impaired renal function, which reduces urine catecholamine excretion and may cause false-negative results
- Failure to collect all urine during the 24-hour period
- Improper specimen storage
- Excessive physical exercise or emotional stress (may raise catecholamine levels)

## DIAGNOSTIC TEST

Abdominal computerized tomography (CT)

**Normal finding**
- Renal parenchyma appears slightly more dense than the liver, but less dense than bone.

**Significant abnormal findings**
- Density differences suggesting renal masses
- Confined, usually detached masses, indicating adrenal tumors

**Interfering factors**
- Patient movement during test may blur images.
- Catheters, surgical clips, or recent contrast studies may impair visualization.

## CUSHING'S SYNDROME

## DIAGNOSTIC TEST

Plasma cortisol

**Normal findings**
*Morning:*
- 7 to 28 mcg/dl
*Afternoon:*
- 2 to 18 mcg/dl

**Significant abnormal finding**
- Elevated plasma cortisol levels

CONTINUED ON PAGE 40

# LAB TESTS

## Interfering factors
• Failure to observe restrictions on diet, medications, or physical activity
• Estrogens (produced during pregnancy or ingested in oral contraceptives) may elevate plasma cortisol levels
• Obesity, stress, severe hepatic or renal disease (may increase plasma cortisol levels)
• Androgens, phenytoin (may decrease plasma cortisol levels)
• Recent (within 1 week) radioactive scan
• Hemolysis from rough handling of specimen

### DIAGNOSTIC TEST
Urine 17-hydroxycorticosteroids (17-OHCS)

## Normal findings
*Men:*
• 4.5 to 12 mg/24 hr
*Women:*
• 2.5 to 10 mg/24 hr

## Significant abnormal finding
• Elevated urine 17-OHCS levels
   *Note:* Levels increase slightly during first trimester of pregnancy. Obese or muscular patients may secrete slightly higher than normal amounts.

## Interfering factors
• Meprobamate, phenothiazines, spironolactone, ascorbic acid, chloral hydrate, glutethimide, chlordiazepoxide, penicillin G, hydroxyzine, quinidine, quinine, iodides, methenamine (may elevate urine 17-OHCS levels)
• Hydralazine, phenytoin, thiazide diuretics, ethinamate, nalidixic acid, reserpine (may suppress urine 17-OHCS levels)
• Failure to collect all urine during the 24-hour period
• Improper specimen storage

### DIAGNOSTIC TEST
Plasma renin activity (PRA)

## Normal findings
*Sodium-depleted, upright, peripheral vein:*
• Ages 20 to 39: 2.9 to 24 ng/ml/hr; mean, 10.8 ng/ml/hr
• Ages 40 and over: 2.9 to 10.8 ng/ml/hr; mean, 5.9 ng/ml/hr
*Sodium-replete, upright:*
• Ages 20 to 39: 0.1 to 4.3 ng/ml/hr; mean, 1.9 ng/ml/hr
• Ages 40 and over: 0.1 to 3.0 ng/ml/hr; mean, 1 ng/ml/hr

## Significant abnormal finding
• Decreased renin levels

## Interfering factors
• Improper patient positioning during test
• Failure to use proper anticoagulant collection tube, to completely fill tube, or to adequately mix the specimen and the anticoagulant
• Failure to chill the collection tube and syringe, or failure to chill and immediately send the specimen to the laboratory. (Either may promote renin breakdown.)
• These factors may increase plasma renin levels: diuretics, vasodilators, and other antihypertensive drugs; oral contraceptives; licorice; sodium intake; severe blood loss; and pregnancy.
• These factors may decrease plasma renin levels: salt-retaining steroid therapy and antidiuretic therapy with vasopressin.

### HYPERPARATHYROIDISM

### DIAGNOSTIC TEST
Serum calcium

## Normal finding
• 8.9 to 10.1 mg/dl (atomic absorption); or 4.5 to 5.5 mEq/liter

## Significant abnormal finding
• Elevated levels (from oversecretion of parathyroid hormone)
   *Note:* A normal or slight decrease suggests secondary hyperparathyroidism.

## Interfering factors
• Androgens, dihydrotachysterol, calciferol-activated calcium salts, progestins-estrogens, thiazides (may elevate levels)
• Ingestion of excessive vitamin D (may elevate levels)
• Acetazolamide, corticosteroids, mithramycin (may decrease levels)
• Long-term laxative use or transfusion of an excessive amount of citrated blood (may decrease levels)

### DIAGNOSTIC TEST
Serum parathyroid hormone (PTH)

## Normal finding
• 20 to 70 µlEq/ml

## Significant abnormal finding
• Elevated levels

## Interfering factors
• Patient's failure to fast overnight
• Hemolysis from rough handling of specimen

# SPECIAL EQUIPMENT

## GETTING ACQUAINTED WITH SPECIAL EQUIPMENT

In recent years, a number of automatic blood pressure monitoring devices have become available. Besides making blood pressure measurement a more exact diagnostic tool by reducing the possibility of human error, these machines save you time.

Of course, blood pressure measurement with a cuff and mercury or aneroid sphygmomanometer is still the usual approach. But under certain circumstances, automatic blood pressure monitors can be valuable tools.

To find out how and when automatic monitors can benefit you and your patients, read the next few pages.

## MONITORING BLOOD PRESSURE WITH THE CRITIKON DINAMAP

The Critikon Dinamap 845, shown here, is ideal for the hospitalized patient who needs frequent blood pressure monitoring but doesn't need an arterial catheter. The monitor provides highly accurate, noninvasive blood pressure and heart rate measurements at intervals as frequent as every 60 seconds.

The Dinamap works by automatically inflating an ordinary pressure cuff placed around the patient's arm. As the cuff deflates, a transducer located in the monitor detects pressure pulsations (oscillations). Having the precalibrated transducer placed inside the monitor contributes to the system's accuracy.

Besides providing systolic, diastolic, and heart rate measurements, the monitor displays mean arterial pressure (MAP) readings after each inflation. MAP is a valuable indicator of the amount of pressure that's available for tissue perfusion.

Dinamap monitor

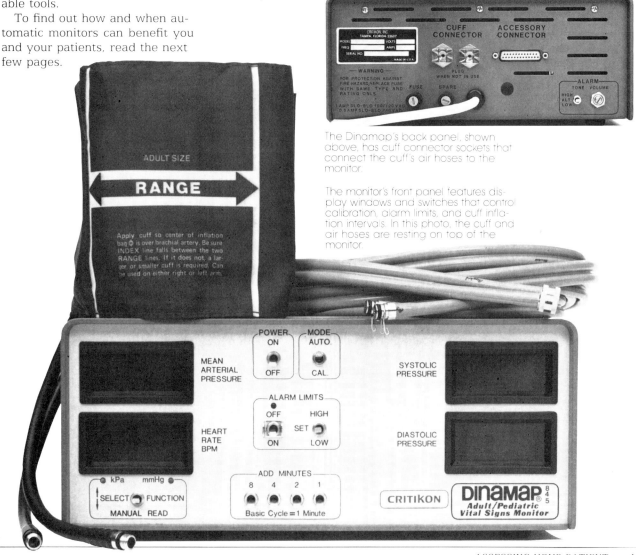

The Dinamap's back panel, shown above, has cuff connector sockets that connect the cuff's air hoses to the monitor.

The monitor's front panel features display windows and switches that control calibration, alarm limits, and cuff inflation intervals. In this photo, the cuff and air hoses are resting on top of the monitor.

# SPECIAL EQUIPMENT

## HOW TO USE THE MEDTEK BPI 420 SYSTEM

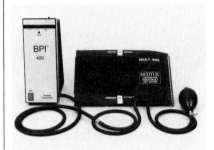

**1** The Medtek BPI 420 system, shown here, permits your patient to monitor his own blood pressure. The system features the BPI 420 unit, occluding/sensing cuff, pressure bulb and AeroMed valve, lockable desk stand/wall bracket, adapter/charger, and extender tubing connector.

Explain the procedure to your patient. Tell him to position the BPI unit in its stand, at his eye level.

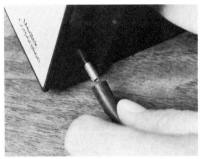

**2** Now, teach him how to attach the tubing to the BPI unit, as shown, and to the unit's extender tubing connector.

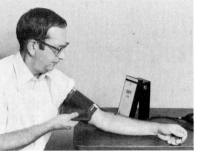

**3** Next, tell your patient to rest his arm on a firm surface level with his heart. Have him extend his arm and apply the cuff. Make sure that the cuff's narrow white band is over the brachial artery and that the cuff fits snugly. The D-ring, or index line, should fall between the two lines on the cuff.

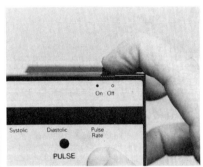

**4** When the cuff's in place, tell your patient to slide the power switch on the top of the unit to ON. As he does, the letters CAL, followed by OCCLUDE, will appear on the screen.

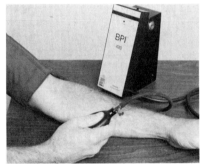

**5** Tell your patient to inflate the cuff by pumping the pressure bulb rapidly until the number on the screen is about 30 mm Hg above his palpatory systolic pressure.

If the letters LO OCC PRESS appear on the screen, tell the patient to pump the pressure bulb once or twice more to increase the pressure.

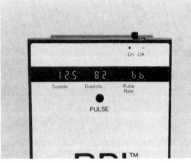

**6** When the patient's artery is occluded, tell him to release the pressure bulb. As he does, the cuff will automatically deflate at the correct rate. Have him record the pressure values and his pulse rate as they appear on the screen, as well as the time and date of the reading.

Finally, show him how to remove the cuff and turn off the unit.

## MONITORING BLOOD PRESSURE AUTOMATICALLY

The Ambulatory Blood Pressure System, featured here, is one of the newest automatic blood pressure monitors available. Manufactured by Instruments for Cardiac Research (ICR), it's currently being evaluated at several hospitals across the country.

The system includes a lightweight, portable monitor that contains a microprocessor to record the measurements; a random access memory (RAM) data pack to store the measurements; a portable operating station for home analysis; an analysis station for hospital analysis; and a detachable battery pack with nonrechargeable alkaline batteries.

The system is simple enough for a patient to use and offers several unique features for both home and hospital use. For the patient's convenience, the system automatically records and stores blood pressure measurements. To facilitate hospital record keeping, it automatically graphs and prints out an analysis of blood pressure data, which could be put in the patient's chart.

To use the system, the patient attaches the monitor to either his belt or a shoulder strap and slips the blood pressure cuff into place. (In the hospital, you'd secure the monitor to the patient's gown.) The microprocessor then records the patient's blood pressure at intervals of 6 to 60 minutes, depending on doctor's orders; displays the digital readings on its mini-screen; and stores them in the RAM data pack.

At the end of the prescribed monitoring period (which is usually 24 hours), the RAM pack is removed from the monitor and placed in either the portable operating station or the analysis station. There, the patient's blood pressure readings are evaluated

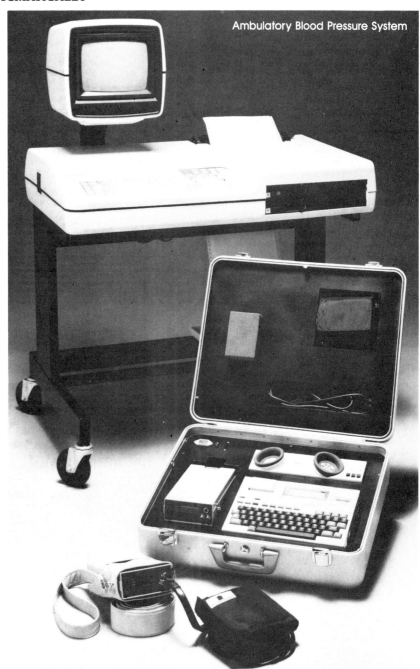

Ambulatory Blood Pressure System

An ambulatory monitoring system like this one permits the health-care team to assess a patient's blood pressure fluctuations as he goes about his daily activities.

for trends, plotted on a graph, and printed out.

The portable operating station can either store blood pressure

information on mini-cassette tapes or transfer it to a central computer. The analysis station stores the information on disks.

# MANAGING HYPERTENSION

Successful hypertension management depends on an important variable—the patient's compliance with his prescribed treatment plan. But gaining your patient's cooperation isn't always easy. After all, he may feel fine. How do you convince him that he must suddenly change the way he thinks, eats, works, and plays? Clearly, you face a challenging task.

This section will help you meet the challenge. In it, we take a close look at the various approaches to hypertension management, from nondrug therapy (including diet changes, exercise programs, and stress reduction) to stepped-care drug therapy. And we offer practical advice on teaching your patient about his condition, motivating him to comply with his treatment plan, and providing ongoing support. To help your patient learn, we've supplied numerous teaching aids that you can copy and give him to take home.

Long-term hypertension management probably won't be easy for your patient. But with teaching, encouragement, and practical advice, you can help your patient control his blood pressure—and improve his prospects for a healthy future.

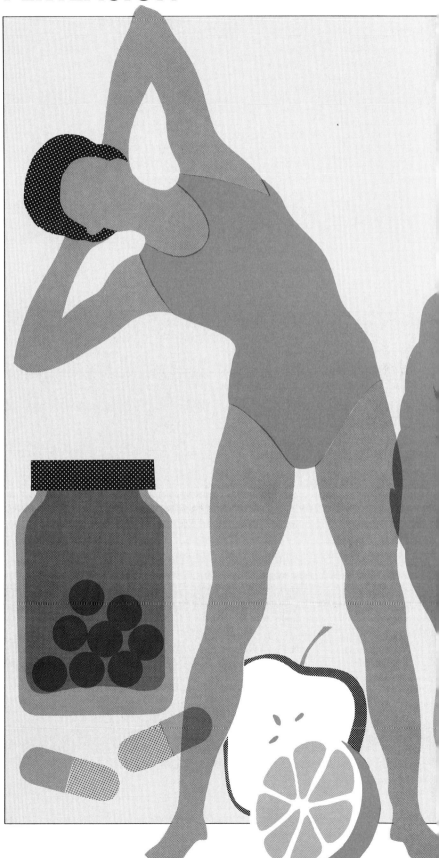

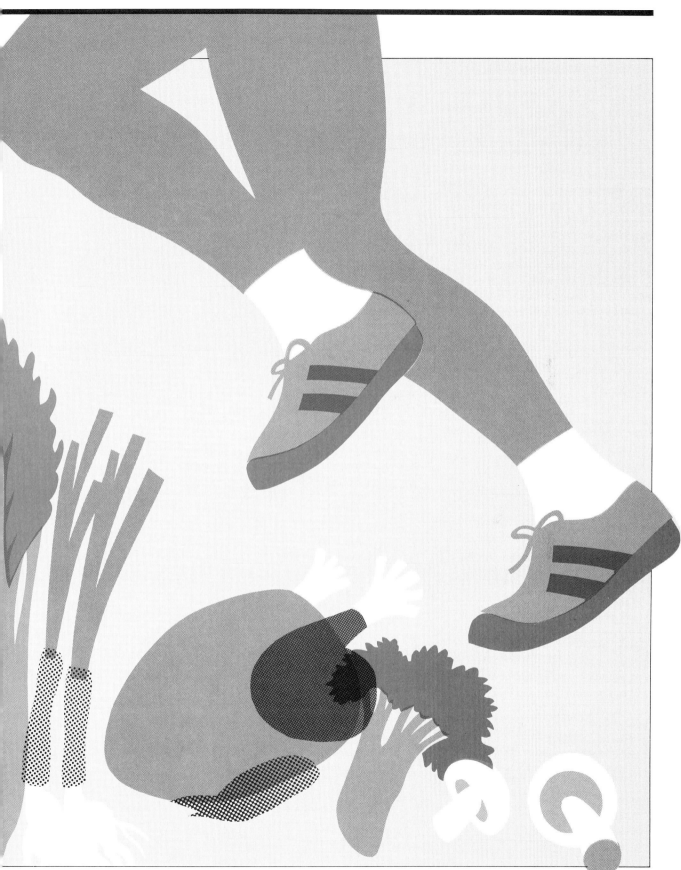

# PATIENT TEACHING

## REACHING YOUR PATIENT: THE FIRST STEP

How do you help someone who may feel fine come to terms with the fact that he has a serious health problem—and persuade him to begin lifelong therapy?

In the case of hypertension, telling your patient about the problem isn't enough. He has plenty of reasons to resist what he hears from you. If he has no symptoms, he may have a hard time believing that a problem exists. The cost of treatment—in money, time, and effort—may make him unwilling to make a commitment. And the fact that his disease is chronic and incurable may discourage him before he begins.

Overcoming these obstacles is no small task. Clearly, patient teaching isn't optional—it's indispensable. In fact, successful hypertension control hinges on making patient teaching an integral, ongoing part of therapy.

Throughout this section, we'll provide teaching tips and aids specific to each facet of antihypertensive therapy. In the next few pages, however, we'll focus on some general guidelines you can use to teach any patient, regardless of his prescribed therapy.

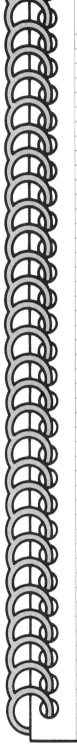

## CRITICAL QUESTIONS

### ASSESSING YOUR PATIENT'S LEARNING NEEDS

What does your patient need to learn to control his condition? To a large extent, that depends on how much he already knows and what life-style changes he needs to make. Begin by assessing his learning needs with an interview. Use the following questions as a guide.

*Note:* Refer to the patient's health history for details about his present health status, medications, and risk factors.

• What does hypertension (high blood pressure) mean?
• What causes it?
• Can you tell when your blood pressure is high?
• What harm does high blood pressure do?
• Can it be cured?
• How do you think treatment will help you?
• How would you describe your eating habits? Do you eat regular, well-balanced meals, or do you tend to snack a lot?
• What are your favorite foods? Do you eat a lot of red meat? Dairy products? Salty foods?
• How much exercise do you get every week?
• How much do you smoke?
• (If your patient is overweight.) Would you like to lose weight? Have you ever tried? If so, how? Were you successful?
• How much alcohol do you drink a day?
• How much coffee do you drink?
• Are you under a lot of emotional stress at work? At home?
• Do you have any vision or hearing problems?
• With whom do you live? Can he (or she) help you follow your treatment plan?
• Would you like to learn how to monitor your blood pressure at home?
• How many grades did you complete in school? (*Remember:* Try to assess your patient's reading ability—never just *assume* that he can read. This assessment affects your choice of teaching tools and methods.)
• Have you ever known anyone with high blood pressure?

## TIPS FOR INTERVIEWING

To get the most out of your interview, you must do more than simply ask the right questions. Asking them in the right way is equally important. Consider the following suggestions and keep them in mind during future teaching sessions.
• Choose a quiet setting. Sit near the patient, at eye level, to help communicate your interest in his remarks.
• Assess your patient's level of understanding, and gear your conversation accordingly. Speak in simple, informal language and avoid medical jargon.
• Ask open-ended questions that encourage more than a *yes* or *no* answer. Listen to his replies without interrupting, and try to document his exact words.
• Be receptive to his concerns—even if they seem relatively unimportant to you. Once you've dealt with *his* concerns, he'll be more willing to answer your questions fully.
• Emphasize the positive and avoid being negative or judgmental. Praise him for seeking help and stress how therapy will benefit him.
• Include the patient's family members (or significant others). Remember, they're part of the patient's support system and play an important role in your patient's compliance.

## SETTING GOALS

Because hypertension is asymptomatic in its early stages, you face a special teaching challenge. Your patient may consider all the life-style changes you propose and conclude, "Why bother? I feel fine!"

Encourage him to establish and maintain a long-term treatment program by taking one step at a time. Help him set long- and short-term goals he can work toward and realistically expect to achieve. By doing so, you avoid overburdening him with too many changes at once—and, in the process, make compliance easier for him.

To make goal-setting effective, don't just tell him what he ought to be working toward. Work with him to identify the goals *he* wants to achieve—and to make sure his goals are within his reach.

**Getting started.** Explain the prescribed therapy in detail. Make sure he understands that all aspects of therapy are important to hypertension control. Remember, some patients assume that adhering to only one aspect of the program—weight reduction, for instance—will do the trick.

Next, ask him to select several short- and long-term goals that seem both worthwhile and attainable to him. A long-term goal might be to maintain blood pressure below 140/90 mm Hg; a short-term one might be to walk six blocks a day, to take all medications on schedule for a week, to lose 3 lb (1.4 kg) in a month—or even to get through an entire Sunday afternoon of football telecasts without opening a bag of potato chips. Your patient will feel better for accomplishing goals he set for himself, and he'll be ready to tackle tougher ones the next time.

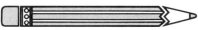

SPECIAL NOTE: Discourage your patient from tackling too much at once. Even if he wants to give up salty foods, quit smoking, and lose 50 lb, he's unlikely to accomplish all three goals immediately. Help him set *realistic* goals—otherwise, he invites failure.

**Involving the family.** Depending on your patient's response to the idea, consider including his family members in goal-setting. If they know what he needs to do and why, they can help him stay on course—and may make changes in the family diet or household routine that'll benefit the whole family.

*Important:* Be sure the patient's family members understand the difference between being supportive and nagging. If you sense negative interactions, encourage the patient and his spouse (or other partner) to role play as you watch. Then, discuss with them the positive and negative behavior this exercise reveals.

**Encouraging compliance.** To help your patient reach mutually agreed-upon short-term goals, you might draw up a list of goals stating his objectives, how to achieve them, and a due date. Make discussion of his progress toward these goals part of your follow-up conferences. You and he might even establish a system of small rewards for meeting the objectives by the due date.

Encourage your patient to call you (or another health-care professional who's following his progress) with questions and concerns that crop up between visits. Consider setting up a regular time for between-visit phone calls.

# PATIENT TEACHING

## TEACHING: SOME METHODS AND TECHNIQUES

Because your patient can't absorb everything he needs to know in only one teaching session, plan to conduct several sessions (the number depends on his particular needs). Then reinforce prior instruction at each successive session.

What's the best way to proceed? That depends on your patient's needs, your time limitations, and the clinical setting and resources. Consider the following options, and use the combination of methods and techniques that works best for you and your patient.

**Teaching techniques.** Make your first session a one-to-one conference to give you a chance to get acquainted with your patient. In later sessions, however, include family members (or significant others). Also, consider including your patient and his family in group teaching sessions. Not only do group sessions help you use your time wisely, but they also provide your patient and his family with guidance and emotional support from others with similar problems.

**Teaching methods.** No matter which format you're using, avoid teaching by rote; in other words,

don't ask your patient to memorize information and repeat it to you. Instead, take a conversational approach, which allows you to fill in information gaps in an informal way.

Introduce new points only after your patient has grasped those you've already made. Encourage him to ask questions whenever he's unsure about something. Take the time to give complete answers. Chances are, your patient will learn more this way than by simply memorizing information.

**Teaching tools.** Groups such as the American Heart Association and the National High Blood Pressure Education Program provide both written and audiovisual teaching aids at varying levels of sophistication. Consider presenting slides or films at group sessions, with question-and-answer periods before and after each session.

Patient-teaching handouts like the one on the following two pages provide the patient with self-care reminders that he can refer to at home. But remember, no handout is a substitute for your personal teaching and learning assessment.

## TEACHING HOME BLOOD PRESSURE MONITORING

No matter what type of antihypertension therapy the doctor prescribes, home blood pressure monitoring may play a part. If your patient is able to monitor his blood pressure, make teaching the proper procedure to him and his family a top priority.

Begin by displaying the equipment and explaining the procedure to the patient and the family member who'll perform the procedure at home. Then, demonstrate the procedure on the patient's arm, while the family member looks over your shoulder. (This enables him to see your demonstration from the same angle he'll work from.) Next, let the family member try. Guide him until he correctly performs the procedure without your help—and feels confident that he can do it alone.

*Important:* Don't expect him to master the procedure at once. Schedule one or more follow-up teaching sessions to make sure he's ready to do it alone.

On pages 49 and 50, we've provided a teaching aid. Give a copy to your patient and his family to help them remember the proper procedure.

## HOME BLOOD PRESSURE MONITORING: HELPING A FAMILY MEMBER AVOID PITFALLS

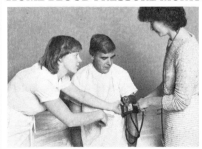

When your patient's family member demonstrates the procedure, watch for errors. For example, if she applies the cuff incorrectly, reinforce your instruction on proper placement.

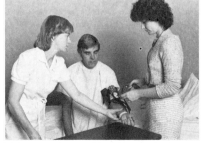

Make sure she positions his arm at heart level. Instruct her to rest his arm on a table or other surface to avoid a false-high reading from isometric muscle contraction.

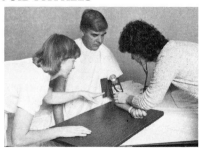

Also stress the importance of reading the gauge at eye level. Encourage her to kneel or crouch, if necessary, for an accurate reading.

## MONITORING BLOOD PRESSURE AT HOME

The nurse has taught you how to take blood pressure readings for a family member. Use these instructions at home, as a reminder.

Measure the patient's blood pressure at these times:

_____.

Notify the doctor if: _____

_____

_____

_____

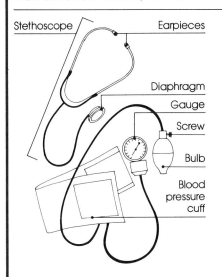

Stethoscope — Earpieces
Diaphragm
Gauge
Screw
Bulb
Blood pressure cuff

**1** To begin, gather this equipment: a stethoscope and a blood pressure cuff with gauge.

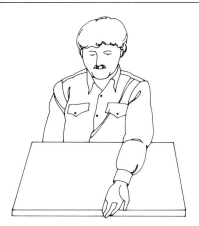

**2** Ask the patient to sit down in a comfortable position and rest his arm on a table, so his arm is level with his heart. (Use the same arm in the same position each time.)

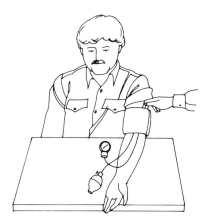

**3** Push up his sleeve and securely wrap the cuff around his upper arm. Wrap it so you can slide only two fingers between it and his arm. Place the gauge where you can easily see it.

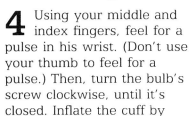

**4** Using your middle and index fingers, feel for a pulse in his wrist. (Don't use your thumb to feel for a pulse.) Then, turn the bulb's screw clockwise, until it's closed. Inflate the cuff by squeezing the bulb rapidly.

Note the reading on the gauge when you no longer feel the pulse. Continue to inflate the cuff until the pressure is 20 points higher than this reading.

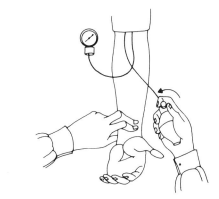

**5** Keeping your fingers at the same spot on his wrist, *slowly* release the air in the cuff by loosening the screw. Now, make a mental note of the reading on the gauge when the pulse returns. This reading is called *palpatory pressure*.

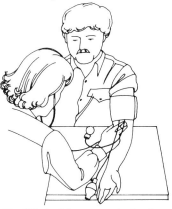

**6** Wait 30 seconds before taking another reading. Then, place the stethoscope's earpieces in your ears. Be sure they're angled forward. Then, place the stethoscope's diaphragm over his brachial pulse (the pulse in the crook of his arm).

CONTINUED

This teaching aid may be reproduced by office copier for distribution to patients. © 1984, Springhouse Corporation

## MONITORING BLOOD PRESSURE AT HOME CONTINUED

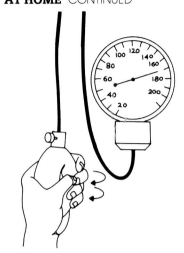

**7** Again tighten the screw and quickly inflate the cuff, until the gauge shows a pressure that's 20 points higher than the *palpatory pressure.*

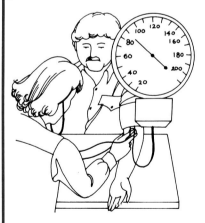

**9** Continue to slowly deflate the cuff, and listen for the beating to stop. As soon as the beating stops, again note the number on the gauge. This is the *diastolic pressure* (the bottom number of a blood pressure reading).

Allow the cuff to deflate quickly and remove it.

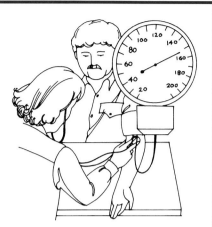

**8** Loosen the screw to allow air to slowly escape from the cuff. Listen for the first beating sound you hear through the stethoscope. When you hear it, note the number on the gauge. This is the *systolic pressure* (the top number of a blood pressure reading).

| DATE | TIME | BP |
|------|------|------|
| 10/22 | 8 PM | 150/90 |
| 10/24 | 8³⁰ PM | 156/86 |
| 10/27 | 7⁴⁵ PM | 150/84 |
| | | |
| | | |
| | | |
| | | |
| | | |
| | | |
| | | |
| | | |
| | | |
| | | |
| | | |
| | | |

**10** Keep a written record of each blood pressure reading you take, including the date and time.

### SELF-MONITORING EQUIPMENT: MAKING A COMPARISON

Teaching a patient's family member or close friend to measure his blood pressure at home is one approach to home blood pressure measurement. But for some patients, self-monitoring is another alternative. For example, a patient may not have any close friends or relatives available to take regular blood pressure readings. Or his spouse or other companion may have a hearing problem that prevents taking accurate readings. And he may prefer the independence that comes with being able to do the procedure himself.

Almost any patient who's willing and motivated can learn to take his own blood pressure. But he'll need your help. Remember, he may think that the procedure is too technical for him to learn. Or he may become frustrated after his first few attempts and feel that he's all thumbs. To help him master the procedure, he'll need help choosing equipment he can handle easily. The following chart offers some guidelines.

When recommending a particular type of equipment, consider your patient's visual acuity, hearing ability, and physical strength. All these factors can interfere with the proper use of certain models (especially standard equipment).

Inform your patient that he can buy equipment at most drug stores or discount department stores. Suggest that he try the equipment before buying anything, to make sure he's comfortable with it. *Note:* Have him pay particular attention to the stethoscope. Inform him that stethoscope earpieces are available in two sizes; encourage him to choose the size that permits him to hear more clearly.

## Portable aneroid sphygmomanometer

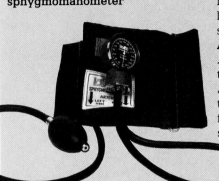

### Description
Nylon cuff with Velcro strips, lightweight stethoscope (not shown), and gauge

### Advantages
*All models:* Lightweight and portable; economical

*Some models:* Extra-large, easy-to-read gauge; cuff with D-ring, for easy one-handed application; stethoscope attached or built into the cuff, for easy one-handed use; self-bleeding deflation valve, which contributes to accuracy; pinless gauge, which signals the need for calibration if the needle fails to rest at zero after deflation

### Disadvantages
*All models:* Stethoscope may not be top quality, so it's unsuitable for a patient with impaired hearing; bulb may be difficult for a weak or arthritic patient to squeeze rapidly; gauge requires regular maintenance and recalibration by the manufacturer.

*Some models:* Without a D-ring on the cuff or attached stethoscope, one-handed cuff application and stethoscope placement may be awkward.

## Portable mercury manometer

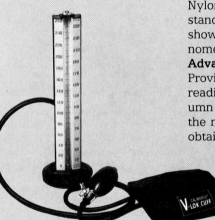

### Description
Nylon cuff with Velcro strips, standard stethoscope (not shown), and mercury-filled manometer

### Advantages
Provides accurate, consistent readings; the wide mercury column may help the patient read the numbers more easily, so he obtains a more accurate reading

### Disadvantages
More expensive; heavier and bulkier, making it inappropriate for patients who must travel frequently; stethoscope may not be top quality; bulb may be difficult for a weak or arthritic patient to squeeze rapidly; mercury (which is toxic in liquid or vapor form) may leak

## Electronic unit

### Description
Electronic cuff, manometer console

### Advantages
*All models:* Easy to use; no stethoscope needed; electronic cuff eliminates human error and is especially appropriate for hearing-impaired patients

*Some models:* Lightweight and compact; cuff with D-ring allows easy one-handed cuff application; automatic inflation and deflation system; large, easy-to-read digital display window; error indicator (for insufficient pressure, improper exhaust speed, low battery voltage). May provide systolic, diastolic, and pulse readings and printouts of all measurements.

### Disadvantages
*All models:* Less accurate than other types; expensive (most types cost much more than standard aneroid equipment); relatively fragile; battery-dependent, must be recalibrated by the manufacturer

*Some models:* May be bulky and not easily portable.

### TEACHING YOUR PATIENT TO MONITOR HIS BLOOD PRESSURE: SOME TIPS

On pages 48 through 50, you learned how to teach a patient's family member to take a blood pressure reading. Teaching the procedure to the patient himself doesn't differ much. But because this one-handed procedure is awkward, consider these tips for making the process easier for him.

• For accurate results, advise your patient to sit down and rest for 15 minutes before taking a measurement.

• Conduct practice sessions with the same type of equipment he'll use at home. If possible, use a double stethoscope to check his ability to recognize Korotkoff sounds. (For help in locating a double stethoscope, consider contacting a local school of nursing.)

• To make it easier for your patient to apply the cuff, show him how to make it into a sleeve and then to slide it onto his arm. If his cuff has a D-ring, tell him to make a sleeve by slipping the

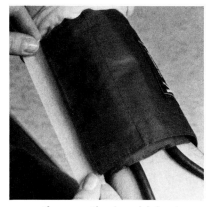

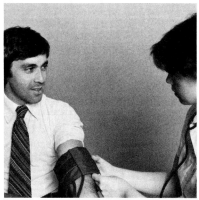

cuff through the ring before putting it on. If the cuff doesn't have a D-ring, he can make a sleeve by fastening the Velcro strips together before applying the cuff, as the nurse is demonstrating above.

• No matter what method he uses, make sure he centers the cuff

correctly over the brachial artery and tightens it properly. Using a piece of tape or a pen, mark the spot on the cuff where he should fasten it (see photo above).

• To help him hold the stethoscope against his brachial artery, suggest that he make two bands out of stretch fabric (such as stretch terry cloth) to apply around his forearm. This will hold the stethoscope securely in place during readings.

• Determine his palpatory systolic pressure, and write it down for him as a reference when he goes home. (Expecting him to determine his own palpatory systolic pressure before each reading is unrealistic; an unsuccessful attempt may frustrate him.) Make sure he understands that he must inflate the cuff 20 to 30 mm Hg above his palpatory systolic pressure before he takes a reading.

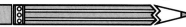

SPECIAL NOTE: If your patient can't manage regular home monitoring, make sure he knows about community blood pressure screening clinics in his area. Remember, even infrequent measurements are better than none at all.

### KEEPING YOUR PATIENT ON TRAC

Expect your patient to have doubts about sticking to his antihypertension therapy. Every time a dietary limitation or other restriction intrudes on his lifestyle, he's likely to ask himself, "Is what I'm going through worth all this trouble?" If you work in a clinic or other outpatient setting, you can encourage him to answer "yes" with follow-up care.

If you're a medical/surgical nurse, you'll probably lose touch with the patient after he leaves the hospital. Nevertheless, you can contribute to his ongoing care by emphasizing the importance of outpatient follow-up care. Encourage him to set up and maintain regular follow-up appointments. If transportation is a problem for him, contact a social service agency for help.

**Outpatient care.** Let's say you're conducting a follow-up visit in an outpatient setting. Start off with an open-ended question, such as "Tell me about your first week on the regimen....How's your family been reacting to it?" Open-ended questions—and attentive listening—communicate your concern for him as a person and reinforce your relationship as partners in his therapy plan.

Follow through with questions about specific problems. If he's keeping a list of goals, go over it with him. Praise him for his successes and accept his failures. Instead of blaming him for shortcomings, ask him what he thinks caused him to fall short, and help him find ways to solve the problem.

**Maintaining long-term contact.** If the patient misses an appointment, make an effort to reach him and reschedule it. Your concern goes a long way toward assuring him that you think the effort is worthwhile.

## DOCUMENTING YOUR PATIENT'S PROGRESS

Before your patient can manage his condition, he has a lot to learn. Documenting his progress is part of your job. Use a chart like this to date and initial his accomplishments.

| Objective: | Session 1 | Session 2 | Session 3 |
|---|---|---|---|
| 1. Defines blood pressure | | | |
| 2. Defines hypertension | | | |
| 3. Defines systolic blood pressure | | | |
| 4. Defines diastolic blood pressure | | | |
| 5. States that the cause of hypertension is unknown | | | |
| 6. States that hypertension is a lifetime condition that can be controlled but not cured | | | |
| 7. States that hypertension is often asymptomatic | | | |
| 8. States the complications of hypertension | | | |
| 9. Defines the following | | | |
|    a. Stroke or cerebrovascular accident (CVA) | | | |
|    b. Heart attack or myocardial infarction (MI) | | | |
|    c. Kidney failure | | | |
| 10. Knows common symptoms of | | | |
|    a. CVA | | | |
|    b. MI | | | |
| 11. States diastolic blood pressure goal | | | |
| 12. States importance of keeping regularly scheduled follow-up appointments | | | |
| 13. Describes effect on blood pressure of the following | | | |
|    a. Smoking | | | |
|    b. Alcohol | | | |
|    c. Sodium | | | |
|    d. Obesity | | | |
|    e. Exercise | | | |
|    f. Emotional stress | | | |
| 14. Identifies the following | | | |
|    a. High-sodium foods | | | |
|    b. Low-sodium foods | | | |
|    c. High-potassium foods | | | |
|    d. High-cholesterol foods | | | |
| 15. Understands that he should | | | |
|    a. Not salt food at the table | | | |
|    b. Cook with half the salt called for in recipes | | | |
|    c. Avoid high-sodium foods | | | |
| 16. Describes the following about prescribed medication(s) | | | |
|    a. Name(s) of medication(s) | | | |
|    b. Dosage | | | |
|    c. Adverse reactions and what should be reported to doctor/nurse | | | |
|    d. What to do if adverse reactions develop | | | |
|    e. Precautions to take while on the medication(s) | | | |
| 17. Understands that doctor may prescribe different drugs or drug combinations | | | |
| 18. Describes ways to remember to take medication(s) | | | |
| 19. Describes ways to reduce stress | | | |
| 20. Describes personal exercise program | | | |
| 21. Maintains blood pressure record | | | |

Patient was given the following pamphlets:

1. _____
2. _____
3. _____
4. _____

Patient was shown the following audiovisuals:

1. _____
2. _____
3. _____
4. _____

# DIET

## CONTROLLING HYPERTENSION NATURALLY

"I have hypertension? But I feel fine!" exclaims Evelyn Wilson, your 42-year-old patient who's recovering from an emergency appendectomy. To her surprise, she's just learned from her doctor that she's hypertensive. Now, she's anxious and upset. Understandably, she's concerned about her condition and worried about the drug therapy she may need.

But Ms. Wilson is lucky. Because her basal blood pressure is 160/94 mm Hg (mild hypertension), her doctor prescribes a nondrug approach to hypertension management. Through proper patient teaching and support, you can help Ms. Wilson control her hypertension naturally, with a low-sodium, low-fat diet. If this approach is successful, Ms. Wilson may be able to postpone drug therapy—or avoid it entirely.

### Why postpone drug therapy?

Although some patients need immediate drug therapy for hypertension control, taking the natural approach can be effective—especially for patients like Ms. Wilson. Increasing evidence shows that about half of all primary hypertension patients can effectively lower their blood pressure with modest sodium restrictions.

Drug therapy, on the other hand, has several drawbacks. First of all, drugs always carry a risk of adverse reactions—and in the case of antihypertensives, these reactions can be debilitating and even life-threatening. What's more, research has not proven that antihypertensive drugs lower morbidity from ischemic heart disease in patients with diastolic pressures below

someone like Ms. Wilson, the risks of drug therapy may outweigh the potential benefits.

**Your role.** As with any therapeutic approach, success hinges on your patient's informed cooperation and participation in the treatment plan. That's where you come in. Part of your job is to help her understand these important points:
• A diet change is serious business, requiring a permanent change in eating habits.
• If diet alone doesn't control her condition, the doctor will probably prescribe drug therapy.
• Even if she needs drug therapy, dietary restrictions will remain an important part of hypertension control.

For details on helping your patient understand and observe dietary restrictions, read on.

## ALCOHOL AND HYPERTENSION

John Somerton is a 52-year-old airline executive who's just learned that he's mildly hypertensive (148/94 mm Hg). His doctor has prescribed a low-sodium, low-fat diet.

While taking Mr. Somerton's dietary history, you learn that he consumes approximately five mixed drinks a day. Because you're aware of a positive relationship between alcohol and hypertension, you're concerned about your patient.

How does alcohol affect your patient's blood pressure? No one is sure, but a relationship seems to exist nonetheless. If a hypertensive patient consumes more than 161 ml of alcohol (about 3 mixed drinks) daily, his already high blood pressure tends to increase. Consequently, his risk of developing coronary artery disease rises.

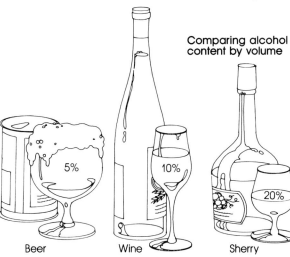

**Comparing alcohol content by volume**

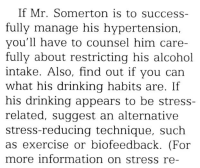

Beer 5%  Wine 10%

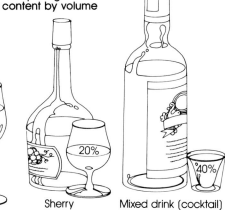

Sherry 20%  Mixed drink (cocktail) 40%

If Mr. Somerton is to successfully manage his hypertension, you'll have to counsel him carefully about restricting his alcohol intake. Also, find out if you can what his drinking habits are. If his drinking appears to be stress-related, suggest an alternative stress-reducing technique, such as exercise or biofeedback. (For more information on stress re-

duction, see pages 64 to 67.)

Offer your patient the following practical advice to help him reduce his intake of alcohol:
• Limit daily alcoholic drinks to the equivalent of about 2 oz (59.1 ml) of 100-proof whiskey.
• Learn to enjoy nonalcoholic beverages, like decaffeinated iced tea or coffee, or have an occasional low-calorie beer.

# SODIUM

## HOW SODIUM AFFECTS BLOOD PRESSURE

Many of us liberally add salt to our food without giving it a second thought. But for a hypertensive patient, this commonly used seasoning is a luxury he can't afford. Here's why.

Nearly half of salt is comprised of sodium, the mineral that causes fluid retention in the body. Fluid retention tends to increase blood volume, which raises peripheral resistance and boosts blood pressure.

By gradually decreasing salt consumption, the patient helps reduce blood volume and peripheral resistance. When arterial blood flow encounters less resistance, blood pressure drops.

## SODIUM CONSUMPTION: HOW MUCH IS TOO MUCH?

When counseling your patient on sodium consumption, keep in mind that avoiding sodium entirely is almost impossible. Sodium is used to process most foods and is a component of many prescription and over-the-counter medications. What's more, a sodium-free diet would be so unpalatable that your patient would eventually stop trying to comply.

The amount of sodium he can safely consume depends on the severity of his condition. If his hypertension is mild, the doctor may restrict his daily sodium intake to 2 to 4 g.

After the doctor's provided guidelines, help your patient plan ways to reduce his sodium consumption. For example, teach him to recognize foods and medications that are high in sodium, so he can eliminate them from his diet. Of course, you'll tell him to avoid such obviously salty foods as potato chips, pretzels, and salted crackers. But also make sure he knows that a food or medication can contain sodium even when it doesn't *taste* salty.

The patient-teaching aid on the next page provides practical guidelines. Carefully review it with your patient. Then, give him a copy to take home.

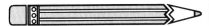

SPECIAL NOTE: Teach your patient to read food labels when grocery shopping to determine an item's sodium content. If a label lists salt instead of sodium, tell him to use the following formula to determine the sodium content in a given amount of salt:

Salt content × 0.4 = sodium content

For example,

200 mg of salt = 80 mg of sodium

## OVER-THE-COUNTER PREPARATIONS: BEWARE OF SODIUM

Be sure to tell your patient about the sodium content of over-the-counter (OTC) oral medications, such as the examples below. Only one dose of some medications may exceed his daily sodium limit.

### OTC PRODUCTS CONTAINING SODIUM

| OTC product | Sodium content |
|---|---|
| Alka-Seltzer | 551 mg/tablet |
| Alka-Seltzer Plus Cold Medicine | 515 mg/tablet |
| Bi So Dol | 157 mg/tsp |
| Cerose-DM | 39 mg/ml of sodium citrate |
| Correctol | 7.82 mg/tablet |
| Di-Gel | 8.5 mg/tsp |
| Maalox Plus | 1.38 mg/tsp |
| Metamucil | 10 mg/tbs |
| Rolaids | 53 mg/tablet |
| Soda Mint Tablets | 88.7 mg/tablet |
| Tussar-2 | 26 mg/ml of sodium citrate |
| Vicks Formula 44 Cough Mixture | 50 mg/ml of sodium citrate |

### THESE OTC PRODUCTS ARE SODIUM-FREE

- Bayer
- Bufferin
- CoTylenol
- Comtrex
- Contac
- Coricidin
- Ecotrin
- Excedrin
- Midol
- Nytol
- Pamprin
- Pepto-Bismol
- Phillips' Milk of Magnesia
- Robitussin-DM
- Sine-Aid
- Sine-Off
- Sominex
- Sudafed
- Triaminic Syrup
- Triaminic Expectorant
- Traminicin
- Tylenol
- Vanquish

## CUTTING DOWN ON SODIUM

To help control your high blood pressure, avoid as many salty foods as possible. This means including more low-sodium foods in your diet and getting out of the habit of adding salt to your food.

Read what follows for some practical advice. Then, review this chart for details on low-sodium foods to enjoy and high-sodium foods to avoid.

• Season foods with herbs and spices instead of with salt.

• Use fresh tomatoes whenever possible for soups and sauces, or use unsalted canned tomatoes, tomato paste, or unsalted tomato juice.

• Season vegetables with vegetable oil, margarine, or approved seasonings, such as parsley or sweet basil.

• Rinse canned foods (including vegetables, tuna, and cottage cheese) under running water to reduce the sodium content.

• Read product labels carefully, keeping in mind that additives are listed in order of greatest quantity. Avoid a product if one of these additives is among the first five listed: salt, sodium benzoate, sodium nitrate, or monosodium glutamate (MSG).

• At restaurants, order boiled, baked, broiled, or roasted foods. Skip gravies, juices, soups, and cheesy dressings.

• Avoid salt substitutes and light salt, unless your doctor approves.

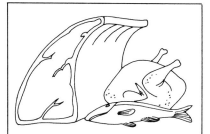

### MEAT
**Low-Sodium Foods:**
Poultry, fresh or frozen fish, veal, lamb, pork, beef
**High-Sodium Foods:**
Sausage, hot dogs, ham, bacon, luncheon meats, salt pork, smoked fish, herring, sardines, canned meat, TV dinners

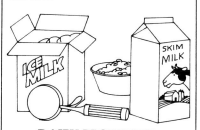

### DAIRY PRODUCTS
**Low-Sodium Foods:**
Skim milk, low-fat cottage cheese, ice milk
**High-Sodium Foods:**
Cheese (especially processed), buttermilk, ice cream

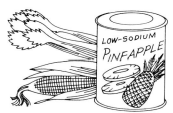

### FRUITS AND VEGETABLES
**Low-Sodium Foods:**
All fresh, frozen, and low-sodium canned fruits and vegetables
**High-Sodium Foods:**
Olives, pickles, sauerkraut, canned vegetables

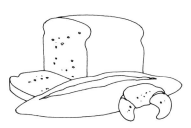

### BREADS AND CEREALS
**Low-Sodium Foods:**
Most commercial and home-made breads
**High-Sodium Foods:**
Salted crackers, pretzels, rye rolls

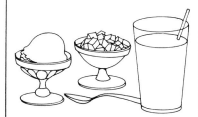

### SNACK FOODS
**Low-Sodium Foods:**
Sherbet, fruit ice, gelatin, fruit drinks
**High-Sodium Foods:**
Potato chips, pork rind, salted nuts, salted popcorn

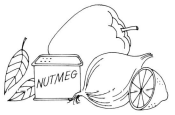

### SEASONINGS
**Low-Sodium Foods:**
Fresh garlic, fresh onion, bay leaf, pepper, dill, nutmeg, rosemary, green pepper, lemon juice
**High-Sodium Foods:**
Salt, garlic or onion salt, bouillon, soy sauce, meat tenderizers, canned soups

# CHOLESTEROL

## CUTTING BACK ON CHOLESTEROL

To help your patient control his hypertension with diet changes, make sure he understands the effects of high plasma cholesterol levels on his health. Review what follows for the background you need.

**Facts about fats.** The body produces a number of fatty compounds called *lipids*. Among the most important are:
• cholesterol, which protects the skin and helps with digestion and hormone formation
• triglycerides, which are formed from carbohydrates and stored in fat cells and adipose tissue as an energy source
• phospholipids, which aid cell membrane formation.

As the name implies, *lipoproteins* are combinations of lipids and proteins; the proportions depend on the lipoprotein type. Two types of lipoproteins are especially important in regulating plasma cholesterol levels.

*High-density lipoproteins* (HDLs) are about 50% protein and 50% cholesterol, triglycerides, and phospholipids. HDLs actually reduce the risk of atherosclerosis by carrying cholesterol away from the peripheral tissues to the liver, which breaks down cholesterol into other lipids.

*Low-density lipoproteins* (LDLs) are about 50% cholesterol; the remaining 50% is composed of protein and lipids other than cholesterol. Although the relationship is unclear, high plasma LDL levels are linked to an increased risk of atherosclerosis and coronary artery disease (CAD).

**Laboratory tests.** To assess your patient's risk of CAD, the doctor may order lipoprotein-cholesterol fractionation. These tests allow him to compare plasma LDL and HDL levels in relation to the total cholesterol level. Normal HDL/cholesterol levels range from 29 to 77 mg/100 ml; higher levels *decrease* CAD risk. Normal LDL/cholesterol levels range from 62 to 185 mg/100 ml; higher levels *increase* CAD risk.

---

*Women tend to have higher HDL levels than men. People who exercise regularly tend to have a more favorable HDL/cholesterol ratio than inactive people.*

---

**Reducing cholesterol consumption.** Dietary restrictions on cholesterol haven't yet been proven to reduce the incidence of CAD (although a low-cholesterol, low–saturated fat diet helps with weight reduction). But remember, your patient's at special risk of atherosclerosis because of vessel damage associated with hypertension. For him, reducing cholesterol intake is a sensible precaution.

The American Heart Association recommends a daily cholesterol limit of 300 mg. To help your patient achieve this goal, teach him to avoid foods high in saturated (animal) fats, which elevate plasma cholesterol and LDL levels. Examples include eggs, whole milk and whole milk products, meat, fat, and bakery products.

Instead, encourage him to eat foods containing unsaturated (vegetable) fats or those that are low in saturated fats. Examples include nuts, margarine, vegetable oils (such as corn, peanut, safflower, and soybean), skinless chicken, and fish.

*Note:* Stress contributes significantly to elevated plasma cholesterol levels. For details on stress reduction, see the information beginning on page 64.

## TIPS FOR SUCCESSFUL LOW-FAT DIETING

Help your patient stick to his low-fat diet by giving him the following advice:
• When shopping, read product labels for fat content (or cholesterol content, if given). Buy only foods made with polyunsaturated or vegetable fats.
• Drink skim milk and use skim milk products.
• Follow your doctor's recommendation for the number of egg yolks you can safely eat each week.
• Limit your intake of beef, ham, and pork. Replace them with poultry, fish, or veal.
• Trim off as much fat from meat as possible before cooking it. Remove all poultry skin.
• Don't fry foods. Sauté food without butter in a nonstick frying pan. Or, use margarine or a nonstick vegetable oil spray.
• If you boil or simmer meat, immediately remove it from the cooking liquid when it's done.
• After preparing soups or gravies, chill them to allow the fat content to congeal; then skim off the fat before reheating and serving.
• Avoid creamy or cheesy sauces.

## KEEPING TRACK OF CHOLESTEROL

To help control the amount of cholesterol in your blood, the doctor wants you to limit your cholesterol intake to less than 300 mg a day. Make sure you stay within this limit by using the following chart, which shows the approximate cholesterol content of some common foods.

| | SERVING SIZE | CHOLESTEROL CONTENT | | SERVING SIZE | CHOLESTEROL CONTENT |
|---|---|---|---|---|---|
| **BREADS** | | | **MEAT** | | |
| biscuit | 1 | 17 mg | bacon | 2 slices | 15 mg |
| bread slice or roll | any amount | 0 mg | beef (lean) | 1 oz | 36 mg |
| French toast | 1 | 130 mg | beef (liver) | 1 oz | 123 mg |
| pancake | 1 | 38 mg | lamb | 1 oz | 37 mg |
| saltine crackers | any amount | 0 mg | pork (ham) | 1 oz | 33 mg |
| sweet roll | 1 | 25 mg | pork (sausages) | 1 oz | 27 mg |
| | | | veal | 1 oz | 38 mg |
| **CHEESES** | | | | | |
| American | 1 oz | 30 mg | **MILK AND DAIRY PRODUCTS** | | |
| cottage cheese | | | butter | 1 tbsp | 30 mg |
|   creamed | 1 cup | 45 mg | egg white | any amount | 0 mg |
|   uncreamed | 1 cup | 16 mg | egg yolk | 1 egg | 245 mg |
| mozzarella | 1 oz | 18 mg | ice cream | ½ cup | 25 mg |
| Muenster | 1 oz | 25 mg | ice milk | ½ cup | 5 mg |
| Parmesan | 1 oz | 25 mg | skim milk | 1 cup | 5 mg |
| provolone | 1 oz | 27 mg | whole milk | 1 cup | 32 mg |
| ricotta | 1 oz | 14 mg | | | |
| Swiss | 1 oz | 28 mg | **POULTRY** | | |
| | | | chicken (light meat with skin) | 1 oz | 22 mg |
| **COOKING OILS** | | | | | |
| lard | 1 tbsp | 12 mg | turkey (light meat with skin) | 1 oz | 23 mg |
| margarine | any amount | 0 mg | | | |
| vegetable oils | any amount | 0 mg | | | |
| | | | **MISCELLANEOUS** | | |
| **DESSERTS** | | | chocolate sauce | any amount | 0 mg |
| angel food cake | any amount | 0 mg | coconut | any amount | 0 mg |
| baked custard | 1 cup | 275 mg | gravy | ¼ cup | 18 mg |
| chocolate cake | 1 slice | 32 mg | low-fat cookies | any amount | 0 mg |
| sherbet | any amount | 0 mg | popcorn (unbuttered) | any amount | 0 mg |
| | | | potatoes | any amount | 0 mg |
| **FISH** | | | white sauce | ¼ cup | 29 mg |
| clams | 1 oz | 13 mg | | | |
| haddock | 1 oz | 23 mg | | | |
| herring | 1 oz | 32 mg | | | |
| oysters | 1 oz | 19 mg | | | |
| salmon | 1 oz | 18 mg | | | |
| scallops | 1 oz | 15 mg | | | |
| shrimp | 1 oz | 57 mg | | | |
| trout | 1 oz | 21 mg | | | |
| tuna | 1 oz | 21 mg | | | |

# EXERCISE

## WHY EXERCISE?

Although nobody's sure *why* exercise reduces hypertension, study after study confirms that it *does.* Blood pressure measurements (and serum cholesterol levels) are lower immediately after brisk activity. Regular exercise eventually results in lower readings all the time. For some patients, exercise does the job so well that the doctor reduces—or even eliminates—drug therapy.

If your patient already exercises regularly, he'll probably need little persuasion to begin an exercise program. If he doesn't, exercising may sound like a lot of work. But when you explain the benefits, he may feel differently. Here's what to say.

Tell your patient that, within a couple of weeks, he'll start to feel more energetic and find his appetite easier to control. With a regular outlet for his energies, he'll probably be better able to cope with stress, too. And he'll have a sense of achievement from taking an active hand in his own treatment.

Although your patient must make the effort himself, you can steer him in the right direction. Read the next few pages for guidelines.

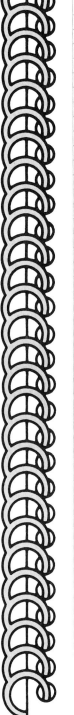

## CRITICAL QUESTIONS

### CAN YOUR PATIENT EXERCISE SAFELY?

Can your patient safely undertake an exercise program? The doctor will consider the patient's medical history, his age, and the rest of his regimen before answering that question. But if mild hypertension is the patient's only health problem, he should have no trouble with an exercise program—as long as he keeps monitoring himself, stays alert for danger signs, and doesn't overdo.

Even so, the doctor may order a treadmill or bicycle stress test to check for underlying complications before allowing him to start an exercise program, especially if he's over age 35. (For details on exercise stress testing, see the NURSING PHOTOBOOK *Giving Cardiac Care.*)

What does the doctor need to know before he recommends an exercise program for your patient? Consider the following questions. If the answer is *yes* to one or more of them, the doctor will modify his recommendation to avoid overstressing the patient.
• Is the patient a heavy smoker?
• Is he more than mildly hypertensive? (If so, the doctor may want the patient to reduce his blood pressure with medication before he starts a regular exercise program.)
• Has he been diagnosed as having unstable angina?
• Has he had a myocardial infarction within the last 3 months?
• Does he show signs of heart failure?
• Does he ever experience chest pain? If so, under what conditions?
• Does he ever experience shortness of breath?
• Is he being treated with ganglionic blocking agents or beta blockers? (Because both of these drug types interfere with normal heart action, they can decrease your patient's tolerance for exercise.)
• Is he diabetic?
• Does he have a chronic respiratory condition, such as asthma?
• Has he recently undergone major surgery?
• Does he ever experience back pain?
• Has he ever injured a knee joint?

# EXERCISE

## MAKING THE RIGHT CHOICE

Advising your patient on an exercise program? Keep in mind that the *type* of exercise he gets is as important as the amount. In fact, he could harm himself by choosing the wrong type, so make sure he understands why you're steering him toward some activities and away from others.

Aerobic (also called dynamic) exercise is the right choice for most patients with hypertension. With an aerobic effort, such as swimming, the muscles move naturally and rhythmically. To supply more oxygenated blood to the muscles as they work, the heart contracts more forcefully and the lungs expand more fully. As a result, the heart muscle becomes stronger and lung perfusion improves.

Systolic blood pressure, which rises only slightly during the workout, may drop 25% or more after aerobic exercise. In time, a regular program of aerobic exercise can permanently lower at-rest blood pressure.

On the other hand, isometric exercise, such as weight lifting, is the wrong choice. Any exercise that involves sustained muscle contraction against resistance—pressing, squeezing, pushing, pulling, lifting—dramatically raises blood pressure. A professional weight lifter may experience blood pressure elevations as high as 450/300 during workouts. And, as any emergency department nurse knows, the strain of even an everyday isometric effort like shoveling snow can quickly overwhelm a weakened cardiovascular system. Isometric exercises build bulk and strength, but they do little to strengthen the cardiovascular system—and that's what your patient with hypertension needs to do.

## HOW TO HELP YOUR PATIENT SET UP A PROGRAM

After the doctor provides guidelines (based on the patient's age, general health, and physical condition), help your patient plan an exercise program.

Encourage him to choose one aerobic activity and stay with it. By sticking to one activity, he'll condition his cardiovascular system more efficiently.

No matter what activity he chooses, he should plan to exercise:
• frequently—at least three times a week.
• for a sustained period—gradually building up to 20 or 30 minutes each time.
• vigorously, so his heart works at 70% to 80% of its maximum rate.

Obviously, the activity should be one he enjoys so it becomes part of his life. It shouldn't be expensive. And, it should be something he can do year-round in some form.

If your patient's not athletic or if he has health problems in addition to his hypertension, walking may be the answer. Suggest that he plan walks where he'll

## CHOOSING THE RIGHT ACTIVITY

Use the examples below to guide your patient toward aerobic exercises and away from isometric ones.

*Note:* Some activities are partly isometric and partly aerobic. For example, when a cyclist leans forward and tightly grips his handlebars as he pedals, his arms are working isometrically while his legs are working aerobically. Alert your patient to this fact, and caution him to keep isometric effort to a minimum.

| AEROBIC EFFORT | ISOMETRIC EFFORT |
| --- | --- |
| Walking briskly | Weight lifting |
| Jogging | Push-ups |
| Running | Waterskiing |
| Swimming | Pulling a heavy golf cart |
| Bicycling | Shoveling |
| Cross-country skiing | Carrying bundles |
| Aerobic dancing | Moving furniture |
| Climbing stairs | Mopping floors |
| Handball | Pushing a vacuum cleaner |
| Racquetball | Opening stuck windows or jar lids |
| Soccer | Sawing hardwood |
| | Judo |
| | Karate |

see new sights every day: a walk around town, for example, is more interesting than six laps around the same block. In bad weather, tell him to walk in a shopping mall during off-peak hours (he can walk faster without crowds around). Remind him to take the stairs between floors. Stress the importance of brisk, *uninterrupted* walking to exercise his heart.

How often should he exercise? At least every other day. After more than 2 days without exercise, he'll start to lose condition.

If he exercises moderately (by brisk walking, for example), he may comfortably maintain a daily schedule. If he exercises vigorously, however, he needs a day's recovery period between exercise sessions. *Important:* Make sure he knows the warning signs of overwork detailed on page 63.

If the doctor has approved routine exercise for your patient, you can show him how to find his target heart rate and check whether he's maintaining that rate during exercise. (For guidelines, see the teaching aid on page 64 and the information below.) Encourage him to work at maintaining his target heart rate for 20 to 30 minutes, with 5 minutes or more of milder work to warm up and 5 minutes to cool down.

As your patient's conditioning improves, his heart will work more efficiently. As a result, it won't have to beat as fast during exertion and its at-rest rate will gradually drop. When it no longer beats at the target rate during exercise, he's ready for more vigorous exercise.

## HOW TO CALCULATE TARGET HEART RATE AND RANGE

To help your patient monitor his exercise program, determine his target heart rate and heart rate range, as explained here. Then, copy the teaching aid on page 64 and write his target rate in the appropriate blank. Give him the aid as a reminder of what you teach him about heart rate monitoring. *Caution:* Always check with the doctor before giving the patient a target heart rate. If the patient has special health problems, the doctor may specify a lower target rate than the following calculations provide.

To calculate target heart rate and target heart rate range, follow these steps:
• Subtract the patient's age from 220. This is his maximum attainable heart rate—the highest rate at which his heart can work. If he's age 40, for example, his maximum heart rate is 180. (This calculation is based on the assumption that a person's heart rate declines by 1 beat/minute for each year he lives.)
• Calculate 75% of his maximum rate to determine his target heart rate. For example, if his maxi-

mum rate is 180, his *target* rate is 135 beats/minute. By maintaining this heart rate during exercise, your patient works his heart at 75% of its capacity—the ideal amount for cardiovascular fitness.
• To determine target heart rate range, calculate the range between 70% and 85% of the pa-

tient's *maximum* heart rate. This calculation provides for the fact that people of the same age may have different resting heart rates. Caution your patient not to exceed his target range. Refer to the chart below for examples of target heart ranges, according to age.

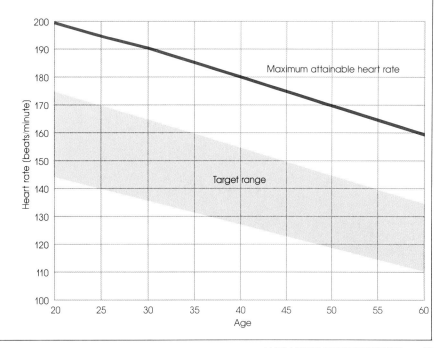

# EXERCISE

## ESTIMATING HEART RATE WITH THE BORG SCALE

As we discussed on page 61, your patient can monitor his heart rate during exercise by simply taking his pulse. But for various reasons, he may not always be able to take a pulse reading—or to get an accurate one. For example, if his heart beats very fast while he's exercising, he may be unable to feel his pulse and accurately count it. Or, if he's bicycling or running, interrupting his exercise to take his pulse may be just a nuisance. At these times the Borg scale, also known as the Rating of Perceived Exertion (RPE) Scale, is useful. Although not as accurate as a pulse rate count, the Borg scale provides a rough estimate that correlates well with the heart rate.

**How to use it.** As shown above, the Borg scale is comprised of numerical values ranging from 6 to 20 with corresponding descriptions. These descriptions reflect levels of exertion ranging from low (very, very light) to high (very, very hard).

To use the scale, the patient first estimates his level of exertion; in other words, how hard he thinks he's working. He then adds a zero to the corresponding numerical value to determine his heart rate when he exercises at this level. For example, if he feels that he's exercising *very hard*, he notes that *very hard* rates 17 on the Borg scale. By adding a zero to this figure, he estimates that his heart rate is 170 beats/minute. Likewise, because *very hard* lies between 16 and 18 on the scale, he estimates that his heart rate is within the range of 160 to 180 beats/minute.

If this exercising heart rate is faster than his target heart rate, he should work less strenuously the next time he exercises. If it's slower than his target heart rate,

### RATING OF PERCEIVED EXERTION SCALE (BORG SCALE)

| | | | |
|---|---|---|---|
| 6 | | 14 | |
| 7 | VERY, VERY LIGHT | 15 | HARD |
| 8 | | 16 | |
| 9 | VERY LIGHT | 17 | VERY HARD |
| 10 | | 18 | |
| 11 | FAIRLY LIGHT | 19 | VERY, VERY HARD |
| 12 | | 20 | |
| 13 | SOMEWHAT HARD | | |

he should work harder.

Of course, the level of exertion your patient aims for depends on his condition and the doctor's guidelines. If he's out of shape, he'll probably start at the *very light* level on the Borg scale and gradually work up to a more strenuous level, as directed by the doctor. If his general health is good and he wants to improve his cardiovascular fitness, he'll try to build up to an exercise that falls within the 12 to 14 rating range on the Borg scale. This range corresponds to 60% to 70% of his maximum heart rate.

No matter what range he aims for, make sure he begins and ends each exercise session with warm-up and cool-down exercises that rate 7 to 9 on the Borg scale.

**Special considerations.** Caution your patient against regarding Borg scale estimates as exact readings. Remind him that they're subjective estimates and that his actual heart rate is influenced by his age, the type of exercise he's doing, and his exercise environment. Because a Borg scale estimate depends on a subjective judgment, he can easily underestimate or overestimate his heart rate.

Familiarize your patient with the Borg scale shown above.

## DOCUMENTING YOUR PATIENT'S PROGRESS

The day you and your patient set up his exercise program, document his weight, body measurements, pulse at rest, target pulse, and blood pressure. Let him know that you (or a clinic or office nurse) will check those numbers at each follow-up visit.

Encourage him to keep his own log of the program. In addition to providing positive feedback, a log serves as a daily record of his progress. In a notebook or in the day blocks of a calendar, have him note each day's exercise. Instruct him to enter his weight, at-rest pulse, and at-rest blood pressure (if he's monitoring his blood pressure at home) once a week only.

Tell your patient to bring his log with him to each follow-up visit, so you can evaluate his progress. Praise him for successes and ask him how he's feeling. Ask him about danger signs—so he doesn't neglect to tell you about a symptom he thought was just part of the aches and pains new exercises may bring. And, of course, keep the doctor aware of your patient's progress.

## WARNING SIGNS: SOME GUIDELINES

Alert your patient to the signals his body may give if he's under too much strain. Some of these signals indicate the body's need for a little rest, but the message of others is, "Go directly to the doctor." Teach your patient to follow these guidelines:

*Call the doctor right away if you feel:*
• an abnormal heart rate: a sudden fluttering, sudden drop in your heartbeat, or skipped beats
• pain in your arms, your throat, or the center of your chest.

*Lie down with your feet up, or sit with your head between your knees, if you feel:*
• faint or dizzy
• confused.
   Talk with the doctor before you exercise again.

*Try a less demanding exercise program, so that you're working to only 65% or 70% of your target rate, if:*
• your heart rate is still high 5 or 10 minutes after your workout.
• you feel nauseous or breathless after exercising.
   Call the doctor if modifying your exercise program doesn't solve the problem.

"Before I began a regular program of aerobic exercise, my health was in real jeopardy. I guess my most dangerous health problem was my hypertension, although I didn't like to admit it at the time. But since I've been exercising regularly, my blood pressure and resting heart rate have declined dramatically. And I really feel the difference, because I have more energy than ever before. Best of all, I know I'm doing something positive to maintain my health for the future."

**Roni Collier**
Aerobics Instructor
North Wales, Pa.

## EXERCISE AND BLOOD PRESSURE CONTROL: A CASE IN POINT

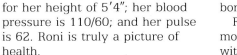

Roni Collier, age 36, is an attractive and energetic mother of two daughters. Roni jogs a little more than 2 miles three times a week and teaches four aerobic exercise classes every week. She weighs 118 lb (54 kg), an ideal weight for her height of 5'4"; her blood pressure is 110/60; and her pulse is 62. Roni is truly a picture of health.

But that picture wasn't always so bright. When she was 21, her doctor diagnosed borderline hypertension but didn't prescribe treatment. Several years later, she became pregnant. At the time, she smoked about two packs of cigarettes a day. Her pregnancy, combined with these two risk factors (smoking and preexisting borderline hypertension) produced a blood pressure rise so steep that she was diagnosed as having severe preeclampsia (pregnancy-induced hypertension, or PIH). Thanks to treatment with a low-sodium diet and a diuretic, however, her pregnancy progressed without further complications. (For more on PIH, see the information beginning on page 100.)

After a normal delivery, Roni's blood pressure dropped to a borderline reading of 138/92. Within 3 months, she lost most of the weight she'd gained during pregnancy. But gradually, over the next few years, Roni gained an additional 27 lb (12 kg). Throughout this time she stopped limiting her sodium intake and continued to smoke heavily. Her blood pressure continued to register at borderline hypertensive levels.

Finally, at age 27, weighing more than 140 lb (64 kg) and still with borderline hypertension, Roni decided that she'd risked her health long enough. She once again changed her eating habits, limiting her sodium and cholesterol intake and eating less fatty meals. In addition, she started jogging and stopped smoking.

A year later, Roni's blood pressure had dropped to 128/84. Still overweight, she joined Weight Watchers and lost 24 lb (11 kg) in 5 months. Since then, Roni's maintained her blood pressure and pulse rate at current levels and she's maintained her ideal weight for the past 8 years.

Of course, the dietary changes helped. But Roni gives the most credit to her active exercise routine. In her own words, "I lowered my blood pressure and stopped smoking through exercise." For a hypertensive patient like Roni, exercise and life-style changes may be the best medicine.

## MONITORING YOUR HEART RATE

Your doctor has given you exercise guidelines. Follow these special instructions: _____

_____

_____.

During exercise, monitor your heart rate as the nurse taught you. Use this teaching aid as a reminder of what you've learned.

Your target heart rate is _____ beats/minute. Try to maintain this rate when you exercise.

How can you check your heart rate? First, get a watch with a second hand. Then, as soon as you stop exercising, take your pulse in one of these two ways:
• Place your index and middle fingers on your wrist just below the thumb, as shown below. (Don't use your thumb to feel for a pulse—it has a strong pulse of its own, which may confuse you.)

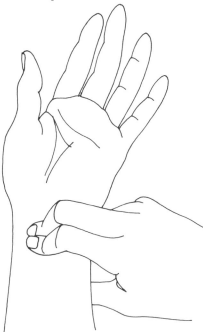

• If you have trouble feeling your wrist pulse, try this: Place your thumb on your collarbone and lay your fingers along the side of your throat, as shown below. You'll feel a strong pulse in your neck.

No matter which method you use, count the pulse beats for 6 seconds; then, add a zero to that figure. This gives you a reliable estimate of your working heart rate for 1 minute. (Don't count your pulse for a whole minute. Because your heart rate slows quickly when you rest, that figure won't be reliable.)

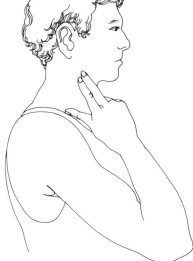

If your working heart rate is 10 beats or more above your target heart rate, don't work so hard the next time. But if your working heart rate is lower than your target rate, work a little *harder* next time. For instance, if you walk, walk faster—or even jog, if the doctor approves.

## STRESS: NOT ALL IN THE MIND

In recent years, interest in reducing emotional and psychological stress has grown to faddish proportions. But don't let this fact mislead you—stress reduction is anything but a frivolous concern. Mounting scientific evidence directly links stress to physical disorders, including hypertension and cardiovascular complications. To understand why, consider the chain of events commonly called the *fight-or-flight* response.

**Fight-or-flight.** When the brain perceives a threat of any sort, it begins to mobilize the entire body for action. The sympathetic branch of the autonomic nervous system releases norepinephrine, and the pituitary gland releases adrenocorticotrophic hormone (ACTH). ACTH, in turn, stimulates the release of corticosteroids—notably, epinephrine and cortisone. Among the results of all this activity are elevated heart rate, increased respiratory rate—and higher-than-normal blood pressure.

Following a fight-or-flight response, the body relaxes and returns to normal. But if stressful circumstances continue, the body tends to stay on alert—and blood pressure remains consistently high.

In addition to high blood pressure, prolonged stress contributes to cardiovascular complications. During the fight-or-flight response, serum cholesterol and triglyceride levels also rise. Triglyceride levels seem to rise in response to *acute* stress, while cholesterol elevations persist following *prolonged* stress. Accumulations of either fatty substance, of course, contribute to the development of atherosclerosis in vessels already damaged by high blood pressure.

And that's not all. As the body prepares itself for danger, the tendency of the blood to clot increases, in preparation for possible injury and hemorrhage. But blood that's quick to clot is also quick to adhere to fatty deposits in the vessels—and so may occlude a crucial vessel, such as a coronary artery.

**Stress and everyday life.** Before initiating the fight-or-flight response, the brain makes little distinction between real physical danger and other threats to well-being. In other words, the body's reaction is similar whether the stress-provoking situation is an impending collision or a heated argument with a co-worker.

---

*Research with animals and studies of people with stressful jobs all point to one conclusion: Stress contributes to hypertension and, in some people, may actually be the cause.*

---

More important than the stressful stimulus itself is the individual's perception and interpretation of the event. For example, if your patient feels secure in his job, a sharp word from a supervisor on a hectic day will roll off his back. But if he's new on the job, that same remark will probably provoke all sorts of anxieties: Is my performance inadequate? Can I handle this job?

Your patient can't do much about many of the stressful situations he encounters each day. But he *can* change the way he reacts to them. And he *must* do so, for his own well-being.

## ACHIEVING DEEP RELAXATION

Although some stress-reducing techniques—biofeedback and self-hypnosis, to name two—require special training, deep relaxation is a technique that your patient can practice himself, with your help. Once he's mastered it, he can use it to enhance other relaxation skills.

To learn deep relaxation, your patient may use one or more of the following techniques. (The teaching aid on page 67 provides yet another alternative.)

**Taped relaxation exercises.** Give your patient a tape recording of a programmed relaxation exercise. Instruct him to listen to it twice daily, preferably not at bedtime. (If he associates the exercise with sleep, he may fall asleep during practice sessions during the day.) Advise him to follow all the instructions on the tape; this encourages him to concentrate on relaxing. With practice, he may be able to relax without the tape.

**Relaxation cues.** This technique is similar to the previous one, except that it doesn't require a tape recording or any other special equipment. As a result, your patient can use it anywhere, anytime.

Tell your patient to select a cue that he associates with deep relaxation. The cue can be anything easily noticed—his watchband, for instance, or a sign on a door near his work place. Tell him to concentrate on the cue as he relaxes. In time, simply looking at the cue may help him relax within minutes.

**Deep breathing.** Teach your patient to breathe rhythmically while staring at a cue object. As he breathes, help him establish a rhythm by counting: for example, "in, 2, 3, 4; out, 2, 3, 4." Keep the pace slow. When he's established a comfortable, relaxing rhythm, urge him to concen-

trate on feeling a little more relaxed with each exhalation. Also tell him to focus on how he feels as he relaxes: weightless, pulsating, tingling, warm, or heavy.

**Imagery.** Tell your patient to think of a place where he usually feels relaxed and carefree—the beach or some other vacation spot, for example. Have him mentally transport himself to that place and concentrate on the details of every sound, sight, smell, and touch he associates with that location.

**Progressive muscle relaxation.** This technique depends on your patient's ability to systematically tense and relax muscle groups throughout his body. Here's how to help him learn this technique:
• Tell him to focus on a particular muscle group. (You might start with the muscles in his hands.)
• Have him tense these muscles.
• After 5 to 7 seconds, signal him to relax the muscles. Urge him to concentrate on the difference he feels between the relaxed and tense states.
• Then tell him to concentrate on another group of muscles (for example, his arm muscles). Signal him to tense them; then to relax them. Continue the procedure until he's tensed and relaxed the muscle groups throughout his body.

To teach a similar technique (sometimes called the Benson response), have your patient progressively relax his muscles from his feet to his head—*without* tensing them first. When he's relaxed, encourage him to perform deep breathing for about 20 minutes.

# STRESS

## UNDERSTANDING BIOFEEDBACK

Your patient may know that relaxing is good for him—but learning to relax is easier said than done. One of the problems, of course, is that he's usually unaware of subtle physical changes that indicate he's beginning to tense up. Biofeedback is a behavioral therapy that solves this problem by putting his conscious mind in tune with these physiologic changes. Once he's mastered a few simple techniques, he can elicit desirable changes and halt undesirable ones at will.

**Biofeedback programs.** Although biofeedback techniques vary according to individual clinics, a therapeutic program may include both of these components:

• mastery of deep relaxation with electronic biofeedback equipment
• continuation of therapy at home, with the patient monitoring his own blood pressure.

In some biofeedback programs, the patient keeps a weekly record of stress-provoking situations and his response to them. By identifying the stressors in his life, he can better learn to manage his responses.

**Who benefits?** Biofeedback is ideal for the mildly hypertensive patient whose condition isn't well controlled by diet. But a patient with more severe hypertension may also benefit from biofeedback, once his condition has been controlled by appropriate drug therapy. Depending on the patient's condition, biofeedback may eventually permit the doctor to reduce or discontinue drug therapy.

Although any stress-reducing technique requires your patient's participation, biofeedback requires special interest and enthusiasm. If your patient's approach to treatment is passive, biofeedback's not for him. But if he wants to actively influence his well-being—and he's willing to spend time learning the necessary skills—consider acquainting him with biofeedback. *Important:* Make sure he understands that biofeedback doesn't *replace* other therapies, such as sodium restriction, weight reduction, and drug therapy.

## ELECTRONIC BIOFEEDBACK: HOW IT WORKS

When your patient asks you to explain electronic biofeedback, can you respond confidently? If not, read this brief overview for details.

To monitor muscle tension, the biofeedback therapist places sensors at the patient's frontalis muscle and wrist. She may also apply sensors at the neck or shoulder, if the patient often feels tense in these areas.

In addition, she applies thermistors to his hands and foot. Why? Consider these facts. As the patient relaxes, sympathetic activity diminishes and the vascular bed dilates. Of course, blood pressure drops—and, as blood supply to the extremities improves, the hands and feet become warmer.

When the equipment's in place, the therapist encourages the patient to relax, using whatever relaxation technique that works best for him; for example, imagery, deep breathing, or progressive muscle relaxation. Electronic signals tell him when he's becoming relaxed.

---

### As a rule, warm hands and feet correspond to relaxation.

---

To help the patient measure his progress, the therapist will help him set physiological goals. For example, the patient may attempt to raise his skin temperature or relax his dominant arm.

With practice, the patient can become skillful enough to relax without electronic feedback. Then, he can easily incorporate brief periods of relaxation into his everyday routine.

## YOUR ROLE

Although a specially trained therapist will teach your patient electronic biofeedback techniques, you'll help prepare him. Follow these guidelines:
• Explain biofeedback—how it works and what he can expect to achieve. Answer his questions.
• Describe the equipment. Assure him that it won't give him a shock.
• Caution him not to expect instant results. Advise him of the need to spend several months training and practicing.
• Tell him to keep the doctor advised of his progress. As the patient's baseline blood pressure drops, the doctor may adjust drug dosages.

### LEARNING HOW TO RELAX

The nurse has explained to you *why* you should relax more to help you lower your blood pressure. This home-care aid will tell you *how* to relax more—on your own, without special equipment. As with any other learning procedure, learning to relax will take practice.

First, choose a slogan that you'll feel comfortable saying each time you practice; for example, "Ease up," or "Slow down." Or, if you prefer, use a short prayer. Then follow the steps shown below.

If you prefer, try this method: Breathe out slowly while concentrating on a particular muscle. Imagine a wave of relaxation starting at the muscle and spreading out to the rest of your body.

No matter what method you choose, do it twice. Then, return to whatever you were doing.

Do your relaxation exercise at least 10 times daily.

---

• Stop whatever you're doing.

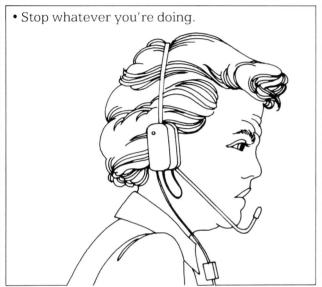

• Smile—openly, if appropriate; otherwise, smile inwardly.

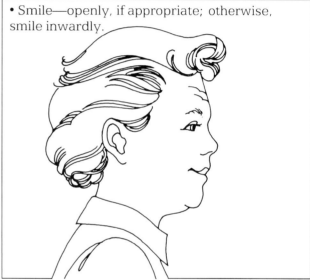

• Say your relaxation slogan to yourself.

SLOW DOWN

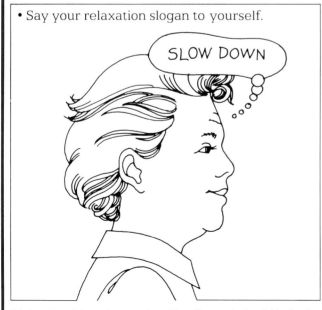

• Take a long, slow, deep breath.
• Breathe out slowly. As you do, think about how relaxed you're feeling.

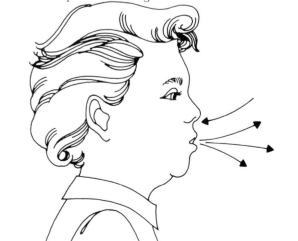

---

# DRUG THERAPY

## DRUG THERAPY: ONE STEP AT A TIME

You're concerned about Muriel Cummings, a 58-year-old housewife who is being treated for hypertension. She's scrupulously maintained a low-sodium diet and reduced her weight by 10 pounds over the past 3 months. Despite her efforts, however, her diastolic blood pressure remains high—above 100 mm Hg. Clearly, conservative measures are not enough to control Ms. Cummings' hypertension. What's the next step?

When conservative treatment fails, expect the doctor to begin antihypertensive drug therapy. To tailor treatment for the patient's needs, he'll probably use a stepped-care approach. This simply means that he'll begin therapy with a diuretic at a low dosage and slowly raise the dosage, as necessary. If the maximum recommended dosage doesn't control her hypertension within about 1 month, he'll add a second hypertensive drug and follow the same protocol. As shown below, this approach consists of four steps. On the following pages, we'll discuss each step in detail.

## TAKING STEPS TO CONTROL HYPERTENSION

For most patients with hypertension, the doctor will begin drug therapy by prescribing a diuretic. Before he proceeds to the next step, he'll rule out poor patient compliance, excessive sodium intake or retention, use of vasoconstricting drugs (such as over-the-counter cold remedies), and secondary hypertension as reasons for the diuretic's failure.

### STEP 4: ADDITIONS OR SUBSTITUTIONS

If the patient is complying with all parts of his regimen but his blood pressure is still uncontrolled, the doctor may proceed to Step 4 of antihypertensive drug therapy. He may order a stronger adrenergic inhibitor (guanethidine sulfate) or a stronger vasodilator (minoxidil) in addition to or instead of the Step 2 drug or Step 3 drug. Or, as an alternative, the doctor may prescribe the angiotensin-conversion inhibitor captopril.

### STEP 3: VASODILATORS

The doctor will prescribe hydralazine hydrochloride or prazosin hydrochloride along with Step 1 and Step 2 drugs. Even if the doctor proceeds to a Step 3 drug because the Step 2 drug caused adverse reactions, he'll continue some dosage of the adrenergic inhibitor. By doing so, he minimizes the vasodilator's effect on the patient's heart rate.

### STEP 2: ADRENERGIC INHIBITORS

The doctor will add a beta blocker, guanabenz acetate, clonidine hydrochloride, or methyldopa if the diuretic alone doesn't control blood pressure. Increase the initial dosage gradually until the drug produces the desired effect. If the dosage reaches the maximum level without producing the desired effect, or if adverse reactions appear, the doctor may add a Step 3 drug.

### STEP 1: DIURETICS

Unless contraindicated, initially give a thiazide (or thiazide-like) diuretic, as ordered. A patient with special problems (for example, renal insufficiency) may need a loop diuretic or a potassium-sparing agent along with the thiazide diuretic.

## PREPARING YOUR PATIENT FOR DRUG THERAPY

Before your patient starts a drug program (or goes from one step to the next), make sure he knows what to expect—and make sure *you* know what concerns he has about treatment. By discussing his concerns with him, you increase his compliance. Keep these points in mind:

• Give your patient a clear picture of how the stepped-care approach works. For example, explain that it starts with the lowest dosage of the mildest drug and is increased only if necessary.

• Tell him about each drug he'll be taking: how it works to lower blood presure, what short-term changes he may notice until his system adjusts, and what adverse reactions it can produce. Tell him about the cost of treatment, too.

• Explore your patient's expectations about the program. If necessary, correct misconceptions.

• Stress that the program won't work without his help. Ask him to tell you or the doctor about any problems he has. Assure him that the doctor can try treatment alternatives if one drug produces unacceptable adverse reactions.

• Reinforce the feeling that you, he, and the doctor are a team working to improve his health. Remind him to make regular follow-up visits. In addition, tell him that he *must* check with you or the doctor before he takes any other medications (prescription or not) or makes any changes in the prescribed regimen.

• Make sure he knows he should inform other health-care professionals—including his dentist—about the drugs he's taking.

## FAILURE TO COMPLY: SOME POSSIBLE REASONS

Many hypertensive patients fail to comply with drug therapy because they experience unpleasant adverse reactions. Which adverse reactions are likely to be most discouraging? A British study (represented by the graph below) suggests some reasons for non-compliance among three groups: those taking a placebo, those taking propranolol hydrochloride (a beta blocker), and those taking bendrofluazide (a thiazide diuretic known in the United States as bendroflumethiazide).

*Note:* If your patient experiences these or any other adverse reactions, urge him to discuss them with his doctor. The doctor can adjust therapy, as necessary.

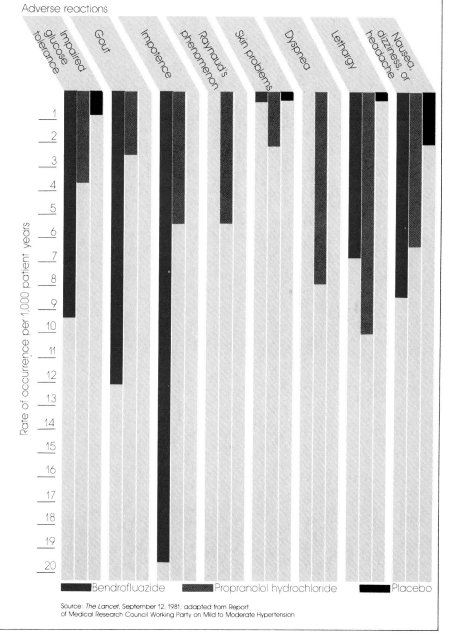

Source: *The Lancet*, September 12, 1981; adapted from Report of Medical Research Council Working Party on Mild to Moderate Hypertension

# DRUG THERAPY

## TREATING BORDERLINE HYPERTENSION: A MODIFIED APPROACH

In the following pages, you'll learn about the widely accepted stepped-care approach to hypertension treatment. But be aware that for a patient with mild or borderline hypertension (diastolic pressure below 95 mm Hg), the doctor may modify the stepped-care approach. Here's why.

**Weighing the risks.** Results from a number of studies suggest that the risk of developing cardiovascular problems in a patient with mild or borderline hypertension is about the same as the average risk among the general population—*unless* the patient has cardiovascular risk factors in addition to hypertension. The most significant cardiovascular risk factors are smoking, hyperlipoproteinemia, and diabetes. For such a patient, eliminating or controlling these risk factors may be more beneficial than lowering his blood pressure with drug therapy.

Another consideration is the fact that drug therapy itself can increase the risk of developing cardiovascular problems in some susceptible patients. One long-term study of patients taking thiazide diuretics (the most common type of Step 1 drug) showed that 30% eventually developed glucose intolerance, another cardiovascular risk factor.

Thiazides can also cause hypokalemia, which can cause dysrhythmias in patients with prior EKG abnormalities. Patients with ventricular irritability are particularly vulnerable.

Finally, thiazides may slightly influence serum lipid levels: serum triglyceride levels may rise 5% to 10%, and serum cholesterol levels may rise up to 5%.

How about other antihypertensive drug types? Beta blockers may reduce high-density lipoprotein (HDL) levels, but their effects on lipids and other lipoproteins is unclear. Other major drug types don't seem to increase the risk of developing cardiovascular problems in most patients.

---

*Drug combination therapy may not be appropriate for a mildly hypertensive patient. But if the doctor does prescribe a drug combination, he may include a diuretic to avoid fluid retention.*

---

**Reversing steps.** With these points in mind, you can understand why the doctor may modify the stepped-care approach for a mildly hypertensive patient. If he decides that drug therapy is indicated, he may avoid exposing the patient to the risks of diuretic therapy by skipping a Step 1 drug altogether. Instead, he may prescribe a Step 2 beta blocker as the initial antihypertensive drug. Although a beta blocker used alone has only mildly antihypertensive effects, it may be all the patient needs. Among patients who may benefit most from beta blockers alone are those who are young; have tachydysrhythmias, ischemic heart disease, or EKG abnormalities; or have high plasma renin levels.

For some patients, however, beta blockers are contraindicated. For these patients, the doctor may order another type of adrenergic inhibitor, such as methyldopa or clonidine hydrochloride. *Note:* Black patients, low-renin hypertensive patients, and the elderly typically respond well to diuretic therapy. For such patients, the doctor may proceed with the traditional stepped-care approach.

## A CASE IN POINT

James Bell, age 35, is an art director for a large advertising agency. Recently, he decided to see his doctor because, as Mr. Bell explained, "Every now and then, my heart would suddenly start beating very fast."

During the first visit, the doctor determined that Mr. Bell had paroxysmal atrial tachycardia (PAT). The doctor also noted that Mr. Bell's blood pressure was elevated (158/94 mm Hg).

At the time Mr. Bell, who has a high-pressure job, was working extra hours and drinking about six cups of coffee a day. Consequently, the doctor advised Mr. Bell to cut back on his caffeine consumption and to reduce his stress through exercise or some other type of stress-reducing activity.

When Mr. Bell returned a week later for a follow-up visit, his heart rate had dropped to 90, but his blood pressure was still high (148/94 mm Hg). So in addition to the previous treatment plan, the doctor prescribed a low-salt diet.

Mr. Bell is scheduled to return in a month for a follow-up check. If his blood pressure is still high, the doctor will likely modify the stepped-care approach and prescribe propranolol hydrochloride (Inderal), a Step 2 beta blocker. Why? Mr. Bell is a young man with a stressful job. Chances are, his high blood pressure and tachycardia stem from excessive catecholamine release related to stress. Because he has no cardiovascular disease that contraindicates beta-blocker therapy, treatment with a beta blocker is an appropriate first step.

# STEP 1

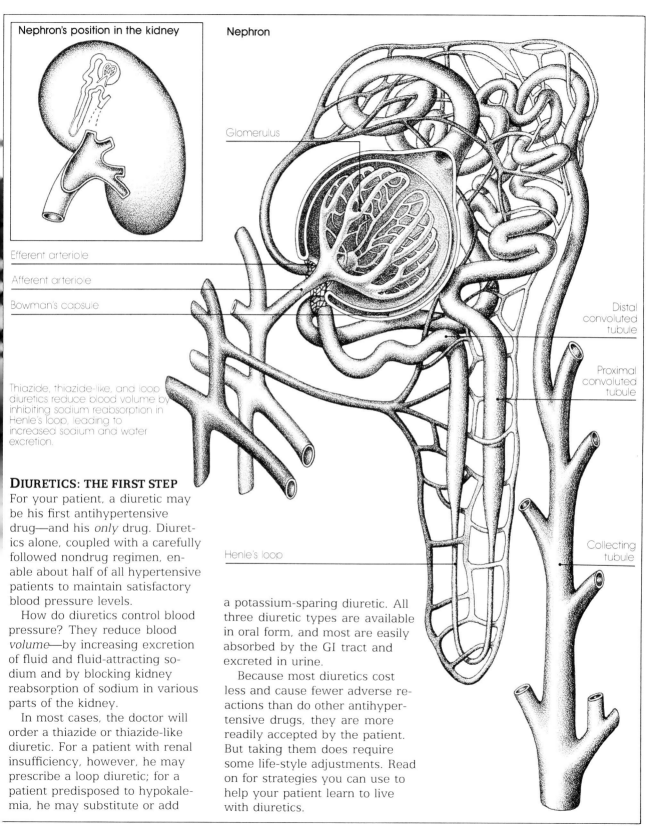

**Nephron's position in the kidney**

**Nephron**

Glomerulus

Efferent arteriole

Afferent arteriole

Bowman's capsule

Thiazide, thiazide-like, and loop
diuretics reduce blood volume by
inhibiting sodium reabsorption in
Henle's loop, leading to
increased sodium and water
excretion.

Distal
convoluted
tubule

Proximal
convoluted
tubule

Collecting
tubule

Henle's loop

## DIURETICS: THE FIRST STEP

For your patient, a diuretic may
be his first antihypertensive
drug—and his *only* drug. Diuretics alone, coupled with a carefully
followed nondrug regimen, enable about half of all hypertensive
patients to maintain satisfactory
blood pressure levels.

How do diuretics control blood
pressure? They reduce blood
*volume*—by increasing excretion
of fluid and fluid-attracting sodium and by blocking kidney
reabsorption of sodium in various
parts of the kidney.

In most cases, the doctor will
order a thiazide or thiazide-like
diuretic. For a patient with renal
insufficiency, however, he may
prescribe a loop diuretic; for a
patient predisposed to hypokalemia, he may substitute or add

a potassium-sparing diuretic. All
three diuretic types are available
in oral form, and most are easily
absorbed by the GI tract and
excreted in urine.

Because most diuretics cost
less and cause fewer adverse reactions than do other antihypertensive drugs, they are more
readily accepted by the patient.
But taking them does require
some life-style adjustments. Read
on for strategies you can use to
help your patient learn to live
with diuretics.

# STEP 1

## PREPARING YOUR PATIENT FOR DIURETIC THERAPY

By teaching your patient what to expect during diuretic therapy, you enhance compliance. Follow these guidelines:

• Prepare him for these initial adverse reactions to therapy: slight weight loss (1 to 2 lb or ½ to 1 kg) within the first few weeks of therapy, increased urine output, fatigue, dry mouth, and possibly postural hypotension. Ask him to report such reactions, but assure him that most will disappear as therapy continues.

• To minimize the effects of postural hypotension, advise him to sit up and stand up slowly, limit alcohol intake, and reduce strenuous activity in hot weather.

• Help him develop a medication schedule that minimizes nocturia. For example, if he takes his diuretic once daily, advise him to take it in the morning. If he takes it twice a day, suggest an early morning/early afternoon schedule.

• Advise your female patient to inform the doctor if she becomes (or plans to become) pregnant while taking antihypertensive drugs.

## LEARNING ABOUT DIURETICS

Familiarize yourself with the three types of antihypertensive diuretics by reading the following chart. All the drugs listed are available in oral form, to permit self-medication.

*Note:* The action, possible adverse reactions, and nursing considerations are identical for thiazide and thiazide-like drugs.

### THIAZIDES

• bendroflumethiazide (Naturetin)
• benzthiazide (Aquapres*)
• chlorothiazide (Diuril)
• cyclothiazide (Anhydron*)
• hydrochlorothiazide (Esidrix, HydroDIURIL)
• hydroflumethiazide (Diucardin)
• methyclothiazide (Aquatensen*, Enduron*)
• polythiazide (Renese)
• trichlormethiazide (Naqua*)

### THIAZIDE-LIKE DRUGS

• chlorthalidone (Hygroton)
• metolazone (Zaroxolyn)
• quinethazone (Hydromox*)

**Action**

Increases sodium and water excretion, which decreases peripheral vascular resistance. Thiazides and thiazide-like drugs also increase urinary excretion of chloride, potassium, and (to a lesser extent) bicarbonate ions. Drug action begins 1 to 2 hours after oral administration.

**Possible adverse reactions**

• Hypokalemia
• Hyperuricemia (gout)
• Hyperglycemia (especially in patients predisposed to diabetes) possibly following the suppression of insulin secretion from diuretic-induced hypokalemia

*Note:* Less common reactions include hyperlipidemia, hypochloremia, metabolic alkalosis, hypercalcemia, azotemia, pancreatitis, rashes, photosensitivity, sexual dysfunction, and blood dyscrasias.

*Not available in Canada

**Nursing considerations**

• Contraindicated in anuria and in hypersensitivity to any thiazide and thiazide-like (sulfonamide-derived) drug. Use cautiously in severe renal disease and impaired hepatic function.

• Use cautiously if patient is also taking digitalis; even asymptomatic hypokalemia may potentiate digitalis, causing digitalis toxicity.

• Use cautiously if the patient's taking lithium; thiazides reduce lithium excretion, possibly causing lithium toxicity. Check serum lithium levels 1 week after any change in thiazide dosage.

• Measure the patient's serum potassium levels before beginning treatment and again 2 to 4 weeks after treatment begins. Monitor for dysrhythmias and advise him to report these signs of hypokalemia: muscle weakness, cramps, fatigue, and GI distress.

• Help patient plan a low-sodium, potassium-rich diet, to prevent or correct hypokalemia.

• To correct severe hypokalemia (serum potassium levels below 3.0 mEq/L), give potassium supplements or add or substitute a potassium-sparing agent (such as spironolactone), as ordered. Asymptomatic mild hypokalemia (serum potassium levels between 3.0 to 3.5 mEq/L) may not require treatment, unless the patient is receiving digitalis, has ischemic heart disease, or has a history of dysrhythmias.

*Caution:* Don't use potassium supplements and potassium-sparing agents together.

• Monitor blood uric acid levels, especially if the patient has a history of gout. As ordered, treat symptomatic hyperuricemia with a drug that promotes uric acid excretion, such as probenecid (Benemid). Asymptomatic hyperuricemia may not require treatment.

• Monitor the patient's blood sugar, especially if he's diabetic; his insulin requirements may need adjustment. If ordered, treat the nondiabetic with severe hyperglycemia with an oral hypoglycemic agent. The doctor may order spironolactone (Aldactone) as an alternative diuretic.

• Explain that the drug will become fully effective within 2 weeks after therapy begins.

• Teach the patient to recognize and report signs of other possible drug side effects, including muscle cramps or weakness, GI changes, skin rash, and joint pain.

## LOOP DIURETICS

• ethacrynic acid (Edecrin)
• furosemide (Lasix)

**Action**

Promotes rapid diuresis by inhibiting reabsorption of sodium and chloride at the proximal portion of the ascending Henle's loop and on proximal and distal tubules. Ethacrynic acid begins to act 30 minutes after oral administration and has a duration of up to 12 hours. Furosemide begins to act in 30 to 60 minutes and has a duration of 6 to 8 hours.

**Possible adverse reactions**

• Same as for thiazide diuretics. In addition, loop diuretics may cause volume depletion and dehydration.

**Nursing considerations**

• Use cautiously if the patient has serum electrolyte abnormalities, since a loop diuretic may cause additional water and electrolyte depletion.

• Loop diuretics are prescribed for patients with renal insufficiency, or in combination with other antihypertensive drugs.

• Use furosemide cautiously if the patient is sensitive to sulfonamide drugs.

• Give cautiously to an elderly patient, because he's especially susceptible to excessive diuresis.

• As with thiazide drugs, monitor the patient for signs of hypokalemia, hyperuricemia, and hyperglycemia. Teach him to recognize the symptoms of these conditions and to report them to his doctor.

• Monitor the patient for oliguria or azotemia. If either condition develops, the doctor may discontinue the drug.

• Teach the patient to store oral furosemide solution in the refrigerator, to ensure the drug's stability.

• Advise him to keep furosemide tablets in a light-resistant container to prevent discoloration. But inform him that discoloration doesn't affect potency.

• Teach him to report these adverse reactions to furosemide: ringing in the ears, severe abdominal pain, sore throat, and fever.

## POTASSIUM-SPARING DIURETICS

• amiloride hydrochloride (Midamor*)
• spironolactone (Aldactone)
• triamterene (Dyrenium)

**Action**

Spironolactone antagonizes aldosterone at the distal tubule, increasing sodium and water excretion but sparing potassium. Amiloride hydrochloride and triamterene aren't dependent on aldosterone for effectiveness. Triamterene inhibits the reabsorption of sodium in exchange for potassium in the distal tubule. When used alone, spironolactone and triamterene become fully effective in 2 to 3 days. Amiloride's effects peak in 6 to 10 hours and last about 24 hours.

**Possible adverse reactions**

• Hyperkalemia
• GI distress
• Blood dyscrasias with triamterene

• Menstrual irregularities with spironolactone
• Gynecomastia with spironolactone
• Mastodynia (breast pain) with spironolactone
• Anaphylaxis with triamterene
• Impotence with amiloride

**Nursing considerations**

• Potassium-sparing diuretics are less potent than both thiazide and loop diuretics. If ordered, administer a thiazide diuretic with the potassium-sparing diuretic to enhance the diuretic effect and reduce the risk of hyperkalemia.

• The doctor may decide to order a potassium-sparing diuretic if the patient has secondary hypertension from hyperaldosteronism, thiazide hypersensitivity, or gout; or if hypokalemia is a special risk (for example, because he's taking digitalis or has ventricular irritability).

• Contraindicated if patient is hyperkalemic. Use with extreme caution if the patient is at risk of hyperkalemia; for example, because of renal insufficiency or insulin dependence with renin deficiency.

• Teach the patient to recognize and report the symptoms of hyperkalemia.

• Tell him to take the drug with or after meals, to reduce GI distress.

• Don't give potassium supplements with potassium-sparing diuretics.

• Protect spironolactone from light.

*Not available in Canada

# STEP 1

## COMPARING THIAZIDE AND THIAZIDE-LIKE DIURETICS

Thiazides and their chemical derivatives, the thiazide-like diuretics, act in similar ways and produce similar effects under most conditions. Duration of action is their greatest difference: some continue acting for up to 3 days, while others work for only 6 to 12 hours. For details, consult the chart below.

Since equal doses of all these diuretics work equally well, the doctor should weigh such patient-compliance factors as cost and convenience before deciding which drug to prescribe.

| Diuretic | Equivalent dose (mg) | Duration of action (hr) |
|---|---|---|
| **Thiazide** | | |
| bendroflumethiazide | 5 | 18 to 24 |
| benzthiazide | 50 | 12 to 18 |
| chlorothiazide | 500 | 6 to 12 |
| cyclothiazide | 2 | 24 to 36 |
| hydrochlorothiazide | 50 | 12 |
| hydroflumethiazide | 50 | 10 to 12 |
| methyclothiazide | 5 | 24 |
| polythiazide | 2 | 24 to 36 |
| trichlormethiazide | 2 | 24 |
| | | |
| **Thiazide-like** | | |
| chlorthalidone | 50 | 48 to 72 |
| metolazone | 5 | 12 to 24 |
| quinethazone | 50 | 18 to 24 |

## DRUG UPDATE

### INDAPAMIDE: A NEW DIURETIC FOR HYPERTENSION MANAGEMENT

The Food and Drug Administration recently approved the clinical use of indapamide (Lozol*), for hypertension management. Although indapamide's mechanism of action isn't fully understood, it apparently lowers blood pressure through its diuretic effect, as well as relaxes peripheral vascular smooth muscle and reduces peripheral resistance. It's indicated for most hypertensive patients, including those with renal impairment.

Indapamide offers two important advantages that may enhance patient compliance:
• It has a relatively long half-life of 18 hours, which requires the patient to take only one daily dose. The usual starting dosage is 2.5 mg daily. But, if necessary, the dosage can be safely increased to 5 mg a day after 4 weeks of therapy.
• Indapamide causes few adverse reactions in most patients. And most of the adverse reactions reported—headache, dizziness, fatigue, and nausea—are mild.

Although uncommon, gout and hypokalemia are also possible adverse reactions to indapamide. The risk of hypokalemia is higher in patients with brisk diuresis or severe cirrhosis and in those on steroid or adrenocorticotrophic hormone (ACTH) therapy. Indapamide may also activate or exacerbate lupus erythematosus.

If the doctor prescribes indapamide for a patient who is already taking an antihypertensive drug, he may cut the other drug's dosage in half—at least initially. In combination with other antihypertensive drugs, indapamide may cause excessive diuresis.

When caring for a patient receiving indapamide therapy, check his serum electrolyte and serum uric acid levels (if ordered), to screen for hypokalemia and gout. If your patient is diabetic or if his health history indicates a predisposition to diabetes, also monitor his serum glucose levels. Indapamide therapy may change his insulin needs or activate latent diabetes.

Indapamide therapy is contraindicated in patients with anuria and in those patients who are hypersensitive to indapamide or other sulfonamide derivatives.

*Not available in Canada

## GUIDE TO POTASSIUM-RICH FOODS

Your doctor has prescribed a water pill (diuretic) to help control your blood pressure. Because this medication may result in the loss of an electrolyte (chemical) called potassium, he may ask you to eat more potassium-rich foods.

The numbers listed below indicate the amount of potassium (in milligrams) found in 100 g (3½-oz serving) of food. All of these foods are high in potassium—but some of them are high in calories, too. So if you're on a low-calorie diet, check with your doctor for further guidelines.

Too little potassium can cause muscle cramps (especially in the legs), muscle weakness, paralysis, and spasms. If you still have these problems after adding potassium to your diet, call your doctor.

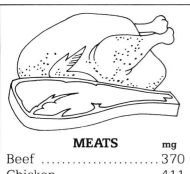

| MEATS | mg |
|---|---|
| Beef | 370 |
| Chicken | 411 |
| Lamb | 290 |
| Liver | 380 |
| Pork | 326 |
| Turkey | 411 |
| Veal | 500 |

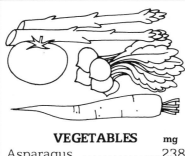

| VEGETABLES | mg |
|---|---|
| Asparagus | 238 |
| Brussels sprouts | 295 |
| Cabbage | 233 |
| Carrots | 341 |
| Endive | 294 |
| Lima beans | 394 |
| Peppers | 213 |
| Potatoes | 407 |
| Radishes | 322 |
| Spinach | 324 |
| Sweet potatoes | 300 |

| FISH | mg |
|---|---|
| Bass | 256 |
| Flounder | 342 |
| Haddock | 348 |
| Halibut | 525 |
| Oysters | 203 |
| Perch | 284 |
| Salmon | 421 |
| Sardines, canned | 590 |
| Scallops | 476 |
| Tuna | 301 |

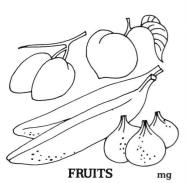

| FRUITS | mg |
|---|---|
| Apricots | 281 |
| Bananas | 370 |
| Dates | 648 |
| Figs | 152 |
| Nectarines | 294 |
| Oranges | 200 |
| Peaches | 202 |
| Plums | 299 |
| Prunes | 262 |
| Raisins | 355 |

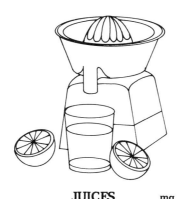

| JUICES | mg |
|---|---|
| Orange, fresh or | 200 |
| reconstituted | 186 |
| Tomato | 227 |

| MISCELLANEOUS | mg |
|---|---|
| Gingersnap cookies | 462 |
| Graham crackers | 384 |
| Oatmeal cookies (with raisins) | 370 |
| Ice milk | 195 |
| Milk, dry (nonfat solids) | 1,745 |
| Molasses (light) | 917 |
| Peanuts | 674 |
| Peanut butter | 670 |

# STEP 2

## HOW ADRENERGIC INHIBITORS WORK

What if diuretics alone don't control your patient's hypertension? Chances are, the doctor will proceed to Step 2 of antihypertensive drug therapy and add an adrenergic inhibitor to the patient's drug regimen. To understand how this drug type helps control hypertension, consider the following facts.

In times of danger or stress, the sympathetic nervous system triggers the release of large amounts of epinephrine and norepinephrine into the systemic circulation. By acting on adrenergic receptors, these hormones produce physiologic and metabolic effects designed to help a person respond appropriately. This process is known as the *fight-or-flight response*. One of its effects include elevated blood pressure.

An adrenergic inhibitor blocks the action of epinephrine and norepinephrine at receptor sites. By doing so, it helps combat those physiologic reactions that tend to elevate blood pressure.

Not all adrenergic inhibitors act on the same receptors, so their indications and effects vary. What's more, they may affect receptors other than those targeted, producing adverse drug reactions. For example, these drugs may affect the central nervous system and cause behavioral changes, such as sedation.

Before prescribing Step 2 therapy, the doctor will rule out these reasons for uncontrolled hypertension: poor compliance with diuretic therapy, excessive sodium consumption, use of vasoconstricting drugs (including some cold remedies), and secondary causes (such as pheochromocytoma).

## ADRENERGIC INHIBITORS AND THE SYMPATHETIC SYSTEM

To fully understand what happens when you administer an adrenergic inhibitor, let's review how the sympathetic nervous system works.

Sympathetic nervous system cells originate in the thoracic ($T_1$) to lumbar ($L_2$) segments of the spinal cord. Impulses sent from the central nervous system travel from the spinal cord along preganglionic nerve fibers to a relay station (called a *ganglion*) outside the spinal cord. From here, the impulses innervate various vital structures; for example, the heart, blood vessels, respiratory tract, liver, urinary bladder, and intestines.

In doing so, they significantly affect the regulation of many body functions. When stimulated, most sympathetic nerves secrete norepinephrine. Norepinephrine, in turn, stimulates receptor sites on the innervated organ.

Within the sympathetic system, two major types of receptors exist: alpha and beta. Alpha receptors, which control vasoconstriction, are located in blood vessels throughout the body. Beta receptors are classified according to location: beta₁ (heart) and beta₂ (bronchioles and peripheral vessels). In the heart, beta₁ receptors increase heart rate and improve myocardial contractility; in the bronchioles and blood vessels, they cause dilation.

Of course, the way a body organ or structure responds to stimulation depends on which receptor predominates. For example, in cutaneous blood vessels alpha receptors predominate. So when norepinephrine is released by the sympathetic system, the alpha receptors are affected, causing these vessels to constrict. By increasing peripheral resistance, this vasoconstriction contributes to hypertension. An alpha blocker, such as phentolamine (Regitine*), blocks this response.

To understand which physiologic responses occur when alpha and beta receptors are stimulated, read the chart below.

| HOW ADRENERGIC RECEPTORS FUNCTION | |
|---|---|
| **Alpha receptors** | **Beta receptors** |
| Vasoconstriction | Vasodilation ($\beta_2$) |
| Pupil dilation | Increased heart rate ($\beta_1$) |
| Intestinal relaxation | Increased myocardial contractility ($\beta_1$) |
| Intestinal sphincter contraction | Intestinal relaxation ($\beta_2$) |
| Pilomotor contraction | Uterus relaxation ($\beta_2$) |
| Bladder sphincter contraction | Bronchodilation ($\beta_2$) |
| | Calorigenesis ($\beta_2$) |
| | Glycogenolysis ($\beta_2$) |
| | Lipolysis ($\beta_1$) |
| | Bladder relaxation ($\beta_2$) |

*Not available in Canada

## PREPARING YOUR PATIENT

To encourage your patient's compliance with therapy, be sure to keep him fully informed about his drug regimen. Stress the importance of taking each drug exactly as prescribed, even when he's feeling well. Tell him to never skip a dose, increase it, or decrease it without asking his doctor. Make sure he understands the possible consequences of noncompliance; for example, rebound hypertension and angina.

In addition, review these general guidelines with your patient:
• Be sure he knows he should inform every doctor (and dentist) who treats him about the drugs he's taking, especially if the doctor plans surgery or may give him an anesthetic.
• Teach your patient about common adverse reactions, such as drowsiness, orthostatic hypotension, and mouth dryness. Tell him that, if he becomes extremely drowsy, he should avoid driving or performing other tasks that require mental alertness and should notify the doctor. The doctor may adjust the dosage or substitute another drug.
• Remind him to avoid sudden rising or prolonged standing. Advise him to stand up slowly to avoid dizziness.
• Tell him to relieve mouth dryness with sugarless gum, sour hard candy, or ice chips.
• Instruct him to call the doctor if he notices any of the following: depression, extreme dizziness, fainting, extreme mouth dryness, nasal congestion, fatigue, headache, numbness, constipation, fever, rash, joint pains, impotence, nightmares, confusion, dark urine, excessive bruising, diarrhea, stomach distress, black stools, weight gain greater than 2 lb (0.9 kg) in 1 day or 7 lb (3.2 kg) in 1 week, chest pains, heart palpitations, or rash.

## NURSE'S GUIDE TO ADRENERGIC INHIBITORS

Adrenergic inhibitors work synergistically with diuretics to reduce blood pressure. You'll administer adrenergic inhibitors in small doses and increase the dosage gradually (as prescribed by the doctor) until the therapeutic effect has been achieved, the maximum dosage has been reached, or adverse drug reactions appear. *Note:* Before the doctor raises the dosage to maximum, he'll consider adding a Step 3 vasodilator.

If the blood pressure goal is reached and maintained with a diuretic-adrenergic inhibitor combination, the doctor may substitute a commercially prepared drug combination to simplify therapy for the patient.

For details on adrenergic inhibitors, refer to the following chart.

---

### CRYPTENAMINE ACETATE (Unitensen Aqueous*)
### CRYPTENAMINE TANNATE (Unitensen*)

**Indications**

To treat mild or moderate hypertension, as well as for treating pregnancy-induced hypertension (preeclampsia)

**Dosage**

Adults: initially, 2 mg P.O. b.i.d., increased at weekly intervals, depending on response. Total daily dosage not to exceed 12 mg.

**Adverse reactions**

Mental confusion, orthostatic hypotension, cardiac dysrhythmias, bradycardia, blurred vision, excessive salivation, unpleasant taste, nausea, vomiting, epigastric burning, hiccups, respiratory depression, bronchial constriction

**Interactions**

• Anesthetic agents may cause additive hypotensive effect.
• Cyclic antidepressants may diminish hypotensive response.

**Precautions**

• Contraindicated in patients with
*Not available in Canada

---

pheochromocytoma.
• Use cautiously in patients with angina, cerebrovascular disease, bronchial asthma, or renal insufficiency and in those taking other antihypertensive agents.
• The range between therapeutic and toxic doses of this drug is narrow. Tell the patient to call the doctor immediately if adverse reactions develop.

---

### ALSEROXYLON (Raudolfin*)
### DESERPIDINE
### RAUWOLFIA SERPENTINA (Raudixin)
### RESCINNAMINE (Anaprel*, Moderil*)

**Indications**

To treat mild or moderate hypertension

**Dosage**

*Alseroxylon*
Adults: initially, 4 mg P.O. daily as a single dose or divided in two doses for 1 to 3 weeks. Maintenance dose: 2 mg or less daily.

*Deserpidine*
Adults: 0.25 mg P.O. t.i.d. or q.i.d. for up to 2 weeks. Maintenance dose: 0.25 mg once daily.

*Rauwolfia serpentina*
Adults: initially and for 1 to 3 weeks thereafter, 200 to 400 mg P.O. daily as a single dose or in two divided doses. Maintenance dose: 50 to 300 mg once daily.

*Rescinnamine*
Adults: initially, 0.5 mg b.i.d. Maintenance dose: 0.25 to 0.5 mg once daily.

**Adverse reactions**

Mental confusion, depression, drowsiness, nervousness, anxiety, nightmares, sedation, parkinsonism, orthostatic hypotension, bradycardia, syncope, mouth dryness, nasal congestion, glaucoma, hyperacidity

**Interactions**

• Monoamine oxidase (MAO) inhibitors may cause excitability and hypertension.

CONTINUED ON PAGE 78

# STEP 2

### Precautions

• Contraindicated in clinically depressed patients and those with a history of depression.

• Use cautiously in patients with severe cardiac or cerebrovascular disease, peptic ulcer, ulcerative colitis, gallstones and in those undergoing surgery. Also use cautiously in patients taking other antihypertensives, anticonvulsants, or cyclic antidepressants.

• Watch the patient for signs of mental depression. Warn him to notify the doctor promptly if he starts having nightmares.

• Instruct the patient to take this drug with meals to increase drug absorption.

### RESERPINE (Serpasil)

#### Indications

To treat mild to moderate hypertension

#### Dosage

Adults: initially, 0.5 mg P.O. daily for 1 to 2 weeks. Maintenance dose: 0.1 to 1 mg daily.

#### Adverse reactions

Mental confusion, depression, drowsiness, nervousness, anxiety, nightmares, sedation, orthostatic hypotension, bradycardia, syncope, mouth dryness, nasal congestion, glaucoma, hyperacidity, nausea, vomiting, gastrointestinal bleeding, pruritus, rash, impotence, weight gain

#### Interactions

• MAO inhibitors may cause excitability and hypertension.

#### Precautions

• Contraindicated in clinically depressed patients and those with a history of depression.

• Use cautiously in patients with severe cardiac or cerebrovascular disease, peptic ulcer, ulcerative colitis, gallstones; in those undergoing surgery; and in those taking other antihypertensive drugs.

• Instruct the female patient to advise the doctor if she becomes pregnant.

• Watch the patient for signs of mental depression. Advise him to notify doctor promptly if he starts having nightmares.

• Instruct him to take this drug with meals to increase drug absorption.

• Have the patient weigh himself daily and notify doctor of any weight gain.

### CLONIDINE HYDROCHLORIDE (Catapres)

#### Indications

To treat primary, renal, and malignant hypertension

#### Dosage

Adults: initially, 0.1 mg P.O. b.i.d. Then, increase the daily dosage by 0.1 to 0.2 mg on a weekly basis. Usual dosage range: 0.2 to 0.8 mg daily in divided doses. Under some circumstances, the doctor may order up to 2.4 mg daily.

#### Adverse reactions

Drowsiness, dizziness, fatigue, sedation, nervousness, headache, orthostatic hypotension, bradycardia, mouth dryness, constipation, urinary retention, impotence

#### Interactions

• Cyclic antidepressants and MAO inhibitors may decrease antihypertensive effect.

#### Precautions

• Use cautiously in patients with severe coronary insufficiency, myocardial infarction, cerebrovascular disease, chronic renal failure, or history of depression.

• Use cautiously if the patient is taking other antihypertensive drugs.

• Warn the patient not to stop the drug without the doctor's permission. Abrupt drug withdrawal may cause rebound hypertension and stroke.

### MECAMYLAMINE HYDROCHLORIDE (Inversine*)

#### Indications

To treat mild to moderate hypertension and uncomplicated malignant hypertension

#### Dosage

Adults: initally, 2.5 mg P.O. b.i.d. Increase by 2.5 mg daily every 2 days. Average daily dose: 25 mg given in three divided doses.

#### Adverse reactions

Paresthesias, sedation, fatigue, tremors, choreiform movements, convulsions, psychic changes, dizziness, weakness, headaches, orthostatic hypotension, mouth dryness, glossitis, dilated pupils, blurred vision, anorexia, nausea, vomiting, constipation, adynamic ileus, diarrhea, urinary retention, decreased libido, impotence

#### Interactions

• Sodium bicarbonate and acetazolamide may increase effect of mecamylamine, causing increased hypotensive effects and toxicity.

#### Precautions

• Contraindicated in patients with recent myocardial infarction, uremia, or chronic pyelonephritis.

• Use cautiously in patients with lower urinary tract pathology, renal insufficiency, glaucoma, pyloric stenosis, coronary insufficiency, or cerebrovascular insufficiency.

• Use cautiously in patients taking other antihypertensive drugs.

• Instruct the patient that this drug's effects are increased by high environmental temperature, fever, stress, or severe illness.

• Warn him against suddenly discontinuing this drug; rebound hypertension may occur. Tell the patient to call the doctor if adverse reactions develop.

• Instruct him to take this drug with meals to increase drug absorption. Tell him *not* to restrict sodium.

• If he develops constipation from

*Not available in Canada

this drug, the doctor may want him to take milk of magnesia. Instruct the patient to avoid bulk laxatives.

## METHYLDOPA (Aldomet)

**Indications**

To treat moderate hypertension. May be used to treat patients with impaired renal function, because it doesn't impair renal blood flow.

**Dosage**

Adults: initially, 250 mg P.O. b.i.d. or t.i.d. in first 48 hours; then increased as needed every 2 days. Dosages may need adjustment if other antihypertensive drugs are added to or deleted from therapy. Maintenance dosage: 500 mg to 2 g daily in two to four divided doses. Maximum recommended daily dose is 3 g.

**Adverse reactions**

Hemolytic anemia, reversible granulocytopenia, thrombocytopenia, sedation, headache, weakness, dizziness, decreased mental acuity, involuntary choreoathetotic movements, psychic disturbances, depression, bradycardia, orthostatic hypotension, aggravated angina, myocarditis, edema, weight gain, dry mouth, nasal congestion, diarrhea, hepatitis, gynecomastia, lactation, rash, drug-induced fever, impotence

**Interactions**

• Norepinephrine, phenothiazines, cyclic antidepressants, and amphetamines may cause hypertensive adverse reactions.

**Precautions**

• Use cautiously in patients receiving other antihypertensives or MAO inhibitors.
• If patient has been on this drug for several months, he may have a positive reaction to direct Coombs' test.
• Instruct the patient to weigh himself daily and to notify the doctor of any weight increase. If sodium and water retention occur, the doc-

*Not available in Canada

tor may prescribe a diuretic.
• Tell patient that his urine may turn dark in toilet bowls treated with bleach.

## ATENOLOL (Tenormin*)

**Indications**

To treat any degree of hypertension. May be used cautiously to treat patients with bronchospastic disorders (such as asthma or emphysema), because drug is relatively cardioselective.

**Dosage**

Adults: initially, 50 mg P.O. daily in a single dose. Dosage may be increased to 100 mg once daily after 7 to 14 days. Under some circumstances, the doctor may order up to 200 mg daily.

**Adverse reactions**

Fatigue, lethargy, bradycardia, hypotension, congestive heart failure, depression, nausea, vomiting, diarrhea, rash, fever

**Interactions**

• Insulin and hypoglycemic drugs (oral) can alter dosage requirements in previously stabilized diabetics.

**Precautions**

• Contraindicated in sinus bradycardia, greater than first-degree heart block, right ventricular failure secondary to pulmonary hypertension, and cardiogenic shock.
• Use cautiously in patients with heart failure and severe peripheral vascular disease.
• Teach the patient to check his pulse before taking this drug. Tell him to hold the drug and call the doctor if his heart rate is slower than 50 beats/minute (or as otherwise directed by the doctor).
• Warn the patient against abruptly discontinuing the drug; this may exacerbate angina and can precipitate myocardial infarction.

*Note:* This drug masks signs of shock and hypoglycemia. But because atenolol and metoprolol tartrate (see following drug listing)

are cardioselective, they may not mask signs of hypoglycemia as completely as some other beta blockers.

## METOPROLOL TARTRATE (Lopressor*)

**Indications**

To treat hypertension. Like atenolol, this drug is relatively cardioselective and may be used cautiously to treat patients with bronchospastic disorders.

**Dosage**

Adults: initially, 50 mg b.i.d. or 100 mg once daily P.O. Maximum dose: up to 200 to 400 mg daily b.i.d. or t.i.d.

**Adverse reactions**

Fatigue, lethargy, bradycardia, hypotension, congestive heart failure, depression, nausea, vomiting, diarrhea, rash, fever

**Interactions**

• Insulin and hypoglycemic drugs (oral) can alter dosage requirements in previously stabilized diabetics.

**Precautions**

• Contraindicated in right ventricular failure secondary to pulmonary hypertension.
• Use cautiously in patients with heart block, congestive heart failure, diabetes, respiratory disease, severe peripheral vascular disease, or in those taking other antihypertensives.
• Teach the patient to take his pulse before giving this drug. Tell him to hold the drug and call the doctor if his heart rate is slower than 50 beats/minute (or as otherwise directed by the doctor).
• Instruct the patient to take the drug with meals to increase drug absorption.

## NADOLOL (Corgard)

**Indications**

To treat hypertension or manage angina pectoris

CONTINUED ON PAGE 80

## NURSE'S GUIDE TO ADRENERGIC INHIBITORS CONTINUED

**Dosage**
Adults: initially, 40 mg P.O. once daily. Dosage may be increased in 40- to 80-mg increments until optimum response occurs. Usual maintenance dose: 80 to 320 mg once daily. In rare cases, doses of 640 mg may be necessary.

**Adverse reactions**
Fatigue, lethargy, bradycardia, hypotension, congestive heart failure, depression, nausea, vomiting, diarrhea, hypoglycemia without tachycardia, rash, increased airway resistance, fever

**Interactions**
• Insulin and oral hypoglycemic drugs can alter dosage requirements in previously stabilized diabetics.
• Epinephrine may cause severe vasoconstriction.
• Indomethacin may decrease antihypertensive effect.

**Precautions**
• Contraindicated in patients with bronchial asthma, sinus bradycardia and greater than first-degree heart block, right ventricular failure secondary to pulmonary hypertension, and cardiogenic shock.
• Use cautiously in patients with heart failure, chronic bronchitis, severe peripheral vascular disease, and emphysema.
• Teach the patient to take his pulse before giving this drug. Tell him to hold the drug and call the doctor if his heart rate is slower than 50 beats/minute (or as otherwise directed).
• Warn him against discontinuing the drug abruptly; this may exacerbate angina and lead to myocardial infarction.
*Caution:* This drug masks signs of shock and hypoglycemia.

---
**PROPRANOLOL HYDROCHLORIDE (Inderal)**
---

**Indications**
To treat hypertension

*Not available in Canada

**Dosage**
Adults: initially, 40 to 80 mg P.O. daily in two to four divided doses or the sustained-release form once daily. Increase at 3- to 7-day intervals to maximum daily dose of 640 mg. Usual maintenance dose for hypertension: 160 to 480 mg daily.

**Adverse reactions**
Fatigue, lethargy, vivid dreams, hallucinations, bradycardia, hypotension, congestive heart failure, depression, nausea, vomiting, diarrhea, hypoglycemia without tachycardia, rash, increased airway resistance, fever

**Interactions**
• Insulin and oral hypoglycemic drugs can alter dosage requirements in previously stabilized diabetics.
• Chlorpromazine and cimetidine inhibit propranolol's metabolism.
• Epinephrine may cause severe vasoconstriction.
• Barbiturates and rifampin may increase metabolism of propranolol.
• Indomethacin may decrease antihypertensive effect.

**Precautions**
• Contraindicated in patients with diabetes mellitus, asthma, allergic rhinitis; during ethyl ether anesthesia; in sinus bradycardia and heart block greater than first degree; in cardiogenic shock; and in right ventricular failure secondary to pulmonary hypertension.
• Use cautiously in patients with congestive heart failure, peripheral vascular disease, or respiratory disease and in those taking other antihypertensive drugs.
• Teach patient to always check his pulse rate before taking this drug. Tell him to hold the drug and call the doctor if his heart rate is slower than 50 beats/minute (or as otherwise directed by the doctor).
• Instruct your patient to take this drug with his meals, in order to increase drug absorption.
*Caution:* This drug masks signs of shock and hypoglycemia.

---
**TIMOLOL MALEATE (Blocadren*)**
---

**Indications**
To treat hypertension and for long-term prophylaxis following acute myocardial infarction

**Dosage**
Adults: initially, 10 mg P.O. b.i.d. Usual maintenance dose: 20 to 40 mg daily. Maximum daily dose: 60 mg.

**Adverse reactions**
Fatigue, lethargy, vivid dreams, bradycardia, hypotension, congestive heart failure, depression, nausea, vomiting, diarrhea, hypoglycemia without tachycardia, rash, increased airway resistance, fever

**Interactions**
• Insulin and oral hypoglycemic drugs can alter dosage requirements in previously stabilized diabetics.
• Indomethacin may decrease antihypertensive effect.

**Precautions**
• Contraindicated in patients with diabetes mellitus, asthma, allergic rhinitis; during ethyl ether anesthesia; in sinus bradycardia and heart block greater than first degree; in cardiogenic shock; and in right ventricular failure secondary to pulmonary hypertension.
• Use cautiously in patients with congestive heart failure, peripheral vascular disease, and respiratory disease and in those taking other antihypertensive drugs.
• Teach the patient to always check his pulse rate before taking this drug. If he detects an extremely fast or slow pulse rate, tell him to hold the drug and call the doctor immediately.
*Caution:* This drug masks signs of shock and hypoglycemia.

## DIFFERENTIATING THERAPEUTIC ACTIVITY

| DRUG | SITE AND MECHANISM OF ACTION | ROUTE | ONSET | DURATION |
|---|---|---|---|---|
| cryptenamine acetate cryptenamine tannate | Stimulates pressor receptors in the heart and the carotid sinus | I.M. I.V. P.O. | 30 to 40 min 2 to 3 min 2 hr | 3 to 6 hr 1 to 2 hr 4 to 6 hr |
| alseroxylon, deserpidine, rauwolfia, and rescinnamine | Peripherally acting; inhibits norepinephrine uptake by depleting its stores | P.O. | Days to weeks | Days |
| reserpine | Peripherally acting; inhibits norepinephrine uptake by depleting its stores | I.M. I.V. P.O. | 2 hr 4 to 60 min Days to weeks | 10 to 12 hr 6 to 8 hr Days |
| clonidine hydrochloride | Centrally acting; inhibits central sympathetic flow | P.O. | 30 to 60 min | 8 hr |
| mecamylamine hydrochloride | Inhibits ganglionic activity by competing with acetylcholine for cholinergic receptors | P.O. | 30 min to 2 hr | 6 to 12 hr |
| trimethaphan camsylate | Inhibits ganglionic activity by competing with acetylcholine for cholinergic receptors | I.V. | Immediate | 10 min after infusion is stopped |
| methyldopa | Centrally acting; activates inhibitory alpha-adrenergic receptors, reducing central sympathetic output | I.V. P.O. | 4 to 6 hr 12 to 24 hr | 10 to 16 hr 24 to 48 hr |
| atenolol | Beta blocker; inhibits response to beta stimulation (also depresses renin output) | P.O. | Days to weeks, depending on dosage | 24 to 36 hr |
| metoprolol tartrate | Beta blocker; inhibits response to beta stimulation (also depresses renin output) | P.O. | Days to weeks, depending on dosage | 12 to 24 hr |
| propranolol hydrochloride | Beta blocker; inhibits response to beta stimulation (also depresses renin output) | I.V. P.O. | 1 to 5 min Days to weeks, depending on dosage | 4 to 6 hr 12 to 24 hr |
| timolol maleate | Beta blocker; inhibits response to beta stimulation (also depresses renin output) | P.O. | Days to weeks, depending on dosage | 12 to 24 hr |
| phenoxybenzamine hydrochloride | Alpha blocker; inhibits response to alpha stimulation | P.O. | Up to 4 days, depending on dosage | 24 to 36 hr |
| phentolamine hydrochloride | Alpha blocker; inhibits response to alpha stimulation | I.M. I.V. P.O. | 2 to 5 min 30 to 60 sec Up to 4 days, depending on dosage | 30 to 45 min 15 to 30 min 24 to 36 min |

# OTHER STEP 2 DRUGS

## NADOLOL: ONE ANSWER FOR NONCOMPLIANT PATIENTS

Nadolol has a longer half-life and duration of action than most other adrenergic inhibitors so it needs to be taken only once a day. This makes it easier for patients (especially the noncompliant ones) to remember. Hence, this beta-blocking drug may help patients maintain therapeutic blood levels.

Consider a starting dose of 40 mg/day typical; this may be gradually increased to 320 mg/day, depending on the patient's condition. Nadolol is available as a 40-, 80-, or 120-mg tablet.

Nadolol shares most of propranolol's adverse reactions and precautions, including the contraindication for patients with asthma (see page 80). Like propranolol, nadolol must be used cautiously in patients with diabetes, congestive heart failure, and emphysema.

Nadolol's longer half-life presents an added problem—drug toxicity. In most cases, bradycardia is the first indicator.

*Note:* Propranolol is now also available in a long-acting form. Atenolol is another beta blocker that offers advantages similar to those of nadolol and propranolol.

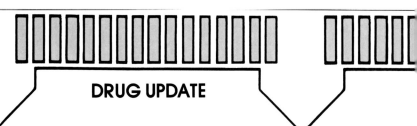

## DRUG UPDATE

### ALTERNATE STEP 2 DRUGS

Guanabenz acetate and pindolol are two relatively new adrenergic inhibitors that the doctor may consider for Step 2 use. Guanabenz is similar to clonidine hydrochloride. Pindolol, like propranolol hydrochloride, is a beta blocker; however, it has several characteristics that distinguish it from other beta blockers. Learn more by reading what follows.

### GUANABENZ ACETATE
#### Wytensin*

**Mechanism of action**
Acts centrally as an alpha-adrenergic receptor agonist

**Dosage**
Adults: 4 mg twice daily. Dosage may be increased daily in increments of 4 to 8 mg every 1 to 2 weeks, to a maximum of 32 mg twice daily.

**Adverse reactions**
Sedation, dizziness, dry mouth, sexual dysfunction

**Special considerations**
• Use cautiously in pregnant and lactating women; the drug's safety for these patients is unproven.
• Use cautiously in combination with drugs that depress the central nervous system, such as phenothiazines, barbiturates, and benzodiazepines.
• Use cautiously in patients with severe heart failure, recent myocardial infarction, cerebrovascular disease, and severe hepatic or renal failure.
• Discontinue therapy gradually to prevent rebound hypertension.

• Warn the patient that the drug may cause drowsiness. Advise him to avoid driving a car or operating other machinery if he experiences this reaction.
• Warn the patient that guanabenz may decrease alcohol tolerance.

### PINDOLOL
#### Visken

**Mechanism of action**
Acts as a nonselective beta blocker and a weak adrenergic agonist. Although its mechanism of action isn't fully understood, pindolol may lower blood pressure by reducing peripheral resistance. Pindolol doesn't reduce cardiac contractility or output as much as do other beta blockers. Because of its special qualities, pindolol is especially helpful for patients with congestive heart failure, asthma, or peripheral vascular disease.

**Dosage**
Adults: 10 mg twice daily alone or in combination with other antihypertension agents. If hypertension is not reduced in 2 to 3 weeks, dosage may be increased daily in increments of 10 mg every 2 to 3 weeks, to a maximum of 60 mg daily.

**Adverse reactions**
Insomnia, dizziness, and fatigue. Less commonly, nightmares, vision disturbances, edema, sexual dysfunction, bronchospasm, and pulmonary fibrosis.

**Special considerations**
• Contraindicated in bronchial asthma, congestive heart failure, cardiogenic shock, second- and

*Not available in Canada

# STEP 3

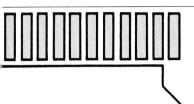

hird-degree heart block, and severe bradycardia.
• Use cautiously in patients taking digitalis and diuretics for congestive heart failure; in those with impaired hepatic and renal function; n those with nonallergic bronchospastic diseases, such as chronic bronchitis and emphysema; and in pregnant women.
• Warn patients, especially those with coronary artery insufficiency, never to interrupt pindolol therapy except under doctor's orders.
• Discontinue pindolol gradually (over 1 to 2 weeks) as ordered; especially in patients with ischemic heart disease (to prevent possible exacerbation of angina or onset of myocardial infarction) and in those who may develop thyrotoxicosis (to prevent thyroid crisis).
• Carefully monitor serum glucose levels in diabetic patients. Pindolol may reduce the amount of insulin the body releases in response to hyperglycemia.
• Monitor the patient for signs of hypoglycemia. Pindolol may interfere with the signs and symptoms of acute hypoglycemia (especially tachycardia and blood pressure changes) and hyperthyroidism (especially tachycardia).
• When used in combination with catecholamine-depleting agents, watch for signs and symptoms of hypotension, such as vertigo, syncope, or postural hypotension, and marked bradycardia.
• Advise lactating women to discontinue breast-feeding.

## VASODILATORS: THE THIRD STEP

As the third step in antihypertensive therapy, vasodilators are lifesavers for patients with peripheral circulatory problems. While diuretics (Step 1) and adrenergic inhibitors (Step 2) work together to reduce blood volume and dampen sympathetic nervous system effects, sometimes this drug combination isn't enough. That's when the doctor may prescribe a vasodilator.

Peripheral vasodilators include hydralazine hydrochloride, minoxidil, and prazosin. These drugs are helpful for hypertensive patients who have vital organ damage. They have limited clinical value for patients with obstructive vascular disease. (Coronary artery vasodilators are another drug type prescribed to abort acute anginal episodes. They're not prescribed for hypertension.)

**How they work.** Normally, arteries are wide enough to accommodate increased blood flow during periods of stress. But when stress triggers the release of large quantities of norepinephrine, the smooth, muscular arteriolar walls constrict, increasing peripheral vascular resistance. Vasodilators relax arterial muscle and improve blood flow.

Because vasodilators widen arteriolar passageways, blood remains in the peripheral veins longer. This reduces venous return to the heart, which, in turn, decreases cardiac output.

At this point, you can see why the doctor prescribes a vasodilator *in addition* to an adrenergic inhibitor. Without the latter drug, a vasodilator triggers this vicious cycle: To maintain cardiac output, the heart beats faster. (Remember: Cardiac output = stroke volume × heart rate.) At the same time, the neuroendocrine response triggers norepinephrine release, which causes vasoconstriction. Vasoconstriction increases peripheral resistance, which improves venous return and boosts blood pressure.

Without an adrenergic inhibitor, the benefits of a vasodilator would be only temporary. An adrenergic inhibitor halts the vicious cycle by slowing heart rate and limiting norepinephrine release.

**When they're indicated.** In most cases, hydralazine hydrochloride (Apresoline) is the vasodilator prescribed. But prazosin hydrochloride may be indicated for some patients. Major indications for these drugs are as follows.
• Hydralazine combats primary hypertension alone or in combination with other antihypertensives. The parenteral form quickly lowers severe blood pressure elevations.
• Prazosin is prescribed for mild to moderate hypertension. Because it acts as an adrenergic inhibitor as well as a vasodilator, it may be used as a Step 2 drug.

## COMPARING SELECTED VASODILATORS

How do three commonly prescribed vasodilators compare? Review the following minichart. For more information on minoxidil, a highly potent vasodilator, see page 87.

| DRUG | ROUTE | ONSET | DURATION |
| --- | --- | --- | --- |
| hydralazine | P.O. | 20 to 30 min | 3 to 8 hr |
| minoxidil | P.O. | 30 min | 24 hr |
| prazosin | P.O. | 2 hr | less than 24 hr |

# STEP 3

## HYDRALAZINE HYDROCHLORIDE (Apresoline)

**Dosage**

Adults: initially, 10 mg P.O. q.i.d.; gradually increase to 50 mg q.i.d. Maximum recommended dosage is 200 mg daily, but some patients may require 300 to 400 mg daily. *Note:* To simplify the patient's regimen, the doctor may order t.i.d. or b.i.d. dosages.

Children: initially, 0.75 mg/kg P.O. daily in four divided doses (25 mg/m² daily). May increase gradually to 10 times this dose, if necessary.

**Adverse reactions**

Peripheral neuritis, headache, dizziness, orthostatic hypotension, tachycardia, dysrhythmias, angina, palpitations, sodium retention, nausea, vomiting, diarrhea, anorexia, rash, lupus erythematosus-like syndrome, weight gain

**Interactions**

• Diazoxide may cause severe hypotension. Use cautiously with hydralazine.

**Special considerations**

• Use cautiously in patients with cardiac disease or in those taking other antihypertensive drugs.
• Teach the patient to recognize signs of lupus erythematosus-like syndrome (sore throat, fever, muscle and joint aches, skin rash). If any of these develop, tell him to call the doctor immediately.
• Instruct the patient to take this drug with meals to increase drug absorption.
• Caution the patient against discontinuing this drug (or any prescribed drug) without his doctor's knowledge.

## PRAZOSIN HYDROCHLORIDE (Minipress)

**Dosage**

Adults: initially, 1 mg given at bedtime, to protect against *first-dose syncope* (severe dizziness or loss of consciousness 30 to 90 minutes following the first dose). Then, 1 mg b.i.d. or t.i.d. May be gradually increased to 20 mg daily; some patients may need dosages of up to 40 mg daily. Usual maintenance dosage range is 3 to 20 mg daily in three divided doses.

**Adverse reactions**

First-dose syncope, dizziness, drowsiness, headache, weakness, depression, orthostatic hypotension, palpitations, blurred vision, dry mouth, vomiting, diarrhea, abdominal cramps, constipation, nausea, and priapism

**Interactions**

None significant

**Special considerations**

• Give prazosin alone or in combination with a diuretic or other antihypertensive drug, as ordered.
• Warn the patient about dizziness and other possible adverse reactions. Advise him to sit or lie down if he feels dizzy, and to stand up slowly. *Note:* As a rule, prazosin causes fewer adverse reactions than does hydralazine.
• Suggest that he relieve mouth dryness with sugarless chewing gum, hard candy, or ice chips.
• Caution him against discontinuing this drug (or any prescribed drug) without his doctor's knowledge.

## USING PRAZOSIN: A CASE IN POINT

Tom Granick, a 66-year-old retired steel worker, is admitted to your unit by his doctor. He went to see his doctor this morning because of increased shortness of breath and leg swelling.

After starting low-flow oxygen using a nasal cannula, you begin your initial assessment. While taking Mr. Granick's history, you discover that he's had hypertension for 5 years and was previously admitted with congestive heart failure (CHF).

His present blood pressure is 180/110. He tells you he takes a water pill twice a day, tries very hard to stay on his special diet, and visits his doctor regularly.

The initial treatment ordered by his doctor has quickly helped relieve Mr. Granick's shortness of breath and edema. His blood pressure, however, remains high. Clearly, diuretic therapy isn't controlling his hypertension.

Because Mr. Granick has a history of CHF, a beta-blocking drug is contraindicated. So, the doctor proceeds to Step 3 drug therapy and orders a stat 1 mg dose of prazosin hydrochloride (Minipress). He tells you that he hopes prazosin's vasodilating effect will lower Mr. Granick's blood pressure and reduce venous return, thus relieving the CHF. (He'll probably also continue the diuretic.)

When you give Mr. Granick his first dose of prazosin, institute these nursing measures:
• Instruct Mr. Granick to stay in bed for the next 2 to 4 hours. Explain that the first dose of this drug may make him feel dizzy.
• Put up the bed's side rails.
• Make sure his call bell is within reach. Caution him against getting up without help.
• Check him frequently.

# STEP 4

## TEACHING YOUR PATIENT ABOUT VASODILATORS

Before you administer any vasodilator to your patient, be sure he understands his disease and the therapy plan the doctor has worked out for him. Because he'll probably be taking more than one medication, help him plan a medication schedule that makes compliance as easy as possible. Then follow these guidelines to be sure he understands all he needs to know about vasodilators:
• Warn him to notify his doctor immediately if he notices any of these adverse reactions: sore throat, fever, muscle and joint aches, or skin rash.
• Caution him that he may experience some light-headedness. He can minimize it by avoiding sudden position changes and by standing up slowly.
• Be sure he understands that he should take his medication exactly as prescribed and continue taking it even after he feels better. Warn him that if he stops taking his medication, his blood pressure will soar out of control again and that uncontrolled high blood pressure may lead to vital organ and eye damage, heart attack, kidney failure, or stroke.

## STEP 4 DRUGS: AN OVERVIEW

If the stepped-care plan's first three steps haven't controlled your patient's hypertension, despite his full compliance, the doctor may proceed to Step 4. In doing so, the doctor has several options. For example, he can:
• replace the Step 2 drug with guanethidine sulfate or guanadrel sulfate, two highly potent adrenergic inhibitors.
• replace the Step 3 drug with minoxidil, a highly potent vasodilator.
• add one of these drugs to the patient's existing regimen.
• replace all antihypertensive drugs *except* the diuretic with captopril.

**How each drug acts.** Like other adrenergic inhibitors, *guanethidine sulfate* (Ismelin) lowers a patient's blood pressure by inhibiting norepinephrine release. In addition, it depletes norepineph-

rine stored in adrenergic nerve endings. But guanethidine causes many adverse reactions, among them orthostatic hypotension. Stress to your patient the importance of telling you about any other medication he's taking, even over-the-counter preparations, because guanethidine interacts with a variety of substances, including alcohol. *Note:* In small doses, guanethidine may be used as a Step 2 drug.

*Guanadrel sulfate* (Hylorel*) is a close relative of guanethidine sulfate that causes fewer adverse reactions. Learn more about this newer drug on page 89.

*Minoxidil* (Loniten*) is a potent vasodilator that many doctors prescribe along with a diuretic and a beta blocker to treat severe hypertension. In addition, it's used for patients with renal hy-

CONTINUED ON PAGE 86

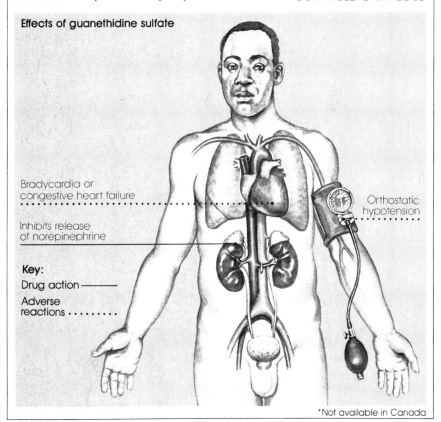

**Effects of guanethidine sulfate**

Bradycardia or congestive heart failure

Inhibits release of norepinephrine

Orthostatic hypotension

**Key:**
Drug action ——————
Adverse reactions ········

*Not available in Canada

## STEP 4 DRUGS: AN OVERVIEW CONTINUED

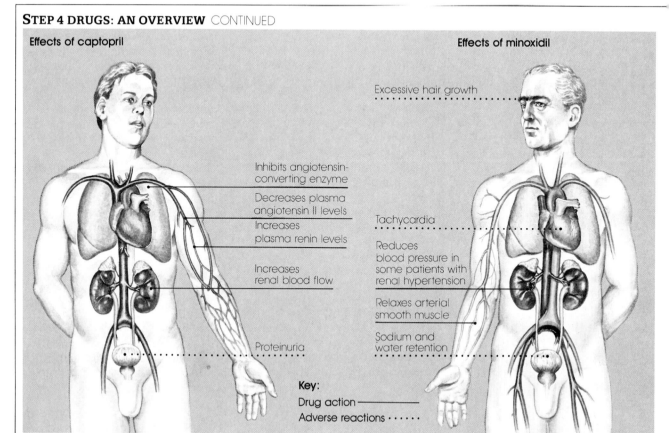

Effects of captopril

- Inhibits angiotensin-converting enzyme
- Decreases plasma angiotensin II levels
- Increases plasma renin levels
- Increases renal blood flow
- Proteinuria

Effects of minoxidil

- Excessive hair growth
- Tachycardia
- Reduces blood pressure in some patients with renal hypertension
- Relaxes arterial smooth muscle
- Sodium and water retention

Key:
Drug action ——————
Adverse reactions · · · · · ·

pertension. Minoxidil relaxes arteriolar smooth muscles to reduce peripheral vascular resistance and lower blood pressure. To prevent sodium and water retention and to minimize tachycardia, a diuretic and adrenergic inhibitor also must be given.

Almost 80% of the patients on minoxidil experience excessive body hair growth (hypertrichosis) as an adverse reaction. (The most common location for hair growth is between the eyebrows.) Usually, this condition peaks 5 to 8 weeks after the initial dose. In 20% to 30% of affected patients, hair growth declines thereafter. Extra hair disappears within 1 to 6 months after stopping minoxidil therapy. Advise your patient that unwanted hair can be controlled with a depilatory or by shaving.

*Captopril* (Capoten\*), a rela-

tively new antihypertensive, inhibits the angiotensin-converting enzyme and prevents the conversion of angiotensin I to angiotensin II. Captopril's anticonversion action decreases plasma angiotensin II and therefore decreases vasoconstriction. Aldosterone secretion is reduced, which increases renal flow and reduces blood pressure. Captopril is nearly always given with a diuretic.

**Captopril: Special considerations.** A possible adverse reaction of captopril is a severe drop in systolic blood pressure following the initial dose. (Reductions greater than 150 mm Hg have been reported.) To lessen the risk of a severe drop, the doctor may take the patient off the diuretic for a week before starting the new drug and instruct the patient to stop restricting his sodium

intake. Both actions increase blood volume and raise peripheral vascular resistance. (If captopril alone doesn't lower the patient's blood pressure, the doctor may then resume therapy with a thiazide diuretic to enhance captopril's effect.)

Warn your patient and his family about possible orthostatic hypotension. If possible, keep him in bed and under close observation for several hours following the first dose.

Throughout therapy, watch for proteinuria and nephrotic syndrome. As ordered, perform white blood cell (WBC) and differential counts before starting therapy, every 2 weeks (or as ordered) for the first 3 months of therapy, and periodically thereafter. Test your patient's urine for protein every month for the first 9 months of therapy (see page 89).

\*Not available in Canada

## GUANETHIDINE SULFATE
### (Ismelin)

**Dosage**

Adults: initially, 10 mg P.O. daily. Increase by 10 mg at weekly to monthly intervals, as ordered. Usual dosage is 25 to 50 mg daily. Some patients require up to 300 mg.

Children: initially, 200 mcg/kg P.O. daily. Increase gradually every 1 to 3 weeks to a maximum of eight times initial dose.

**Adverse reactions**

Dizziness, weakness, syncope, orthostatic hypotension, bradycardia, congestive heart failure, dysrhythmias, nasal stuffiness, mouth dryness, diarrhea, edema, weight gain, inhibition of ejaculation

**Precautions**

• Contraindicated in patients with pheochromocytoma.

• Use cautiously in patients with severe cardiac disease, recent MI, cerebrovascular disease, peptic ulcer, impaired renal function, bronchial asthma, or in those taking other antihypertensives.

**Nursing consideration**

• Discontinue drug 2 to 3 weeks before elective surgery to reduce the risk of vascular collapse and cardiac arrest during anesthesia.

## MINOXIDIL (Loniten*)

**Dosage**

Adults: initially 5 mg P.O. as a single dose. Effective dosage range is usually 10 to 40 mg/day given b.i.d. Maximum dosage is 100 mg/day.

Children (under 12 years): 0.2 mg/kg as a single daily dose. Usual dosage range is 0.25 to 1 mg/kg/day. Maximum daily dosage is 50 mg.

**Adverse reactions**

Edema, tachycardia, pericardial effusion and tamponade, congestive heart failure, EKG changes, hypertrichosis, breast tenderness

*Not available in Canada

**Precautions**

• Contraindicated in patients with pheochromocytoma.

• Use cautiously with guanethidine; may cause severe orthostatic hypotension.

**Nursing considerations**

• Minoxidil is a potent vasodilator; it's indicated only when other antihypertensives have failed.

• Advise the patient that unwanted hair can be controlled with a depilatory or by shaving. Assure him that extra hair will disappear within 1 to 6 months of discontinuing minoxidil therapy.

• Instruct the patient not to discontinue the drug without the doctor's consent.

• Inform the patient that he may experience swelling. Tell him to notify the doctor if he suddenly gains weight.

• Be aware that this drug is usually prescribed with a beta-blocking drug to control tachycardia and a diuretic to counteract fluid retention. Make sure the patient complies with the total regimen.

• Be sure that your patient receives the patient package insert (PPI) and reads it thoroughly. Also, provide an oral explanation.

## CAPTOPRIL (Capoten*)

**Dosage**

Adults: initially, 25 mg t.i.d. If blood pressure isn't satisfactorily controlled in 1 to 2 weeks, dosage may be increased to 50 mg t.i.d. If not satisfactorily controlled after another 1 to 2 weeks, a diuretic should be added to the regimen. If further blood pressure reduction is necessary, the dosage may be raised as high as 150 mg t.i.d. while continuing the diuretic. Maximum dose is 450 mg/day.

**Adverse reactions**

Leukopenia, agranulocytosis, pancytopenia, dizziness, fainting, tachycardia, hypotension, angina pectoris, congestive heart failure, loss of taste (dysgeusia), anorexia, proteinuria, nephrotic syndrome, membranous glomerulopathy, renal failure, urinary frequency, urticarial rash, maculopapular rash, pruritus, fever, angioedema of face and extremities, transient increases in liver enzymes

**Precautions**

• Use cautiously in patients with impaired renal function or serious autoimmune disease (particularly systemic lupus erythematosus) or in those who have been exposed to other drugs known to affect white cell counts or immune response.

**Nursing considerations**

• Be aware that proteinuria and nephrotic syndrome may occur in a patient who is on captopril therapy. If a patient develops persistent proteinuria, or proteinuria that exceeds 1 g/day, suggest having his captopril therapy reevaluated.

• Obtain blood specimen for WBC and differential counts before starting treatment, then after every 2 weeks for the first 3 months of therapy, and periodically thereafter.

• Advise the patient to report any sign of infection, such as a sore throat or fever.

• Although captopril can be used alone, be aware that its beneficial effects increase when a thiazide diuretic is added.

• Advise the patient to avoid sudden position changes, since the drug may cause orthostatic hypotension.

• Inform the patient that taste sensation may be impaired.

• Instruct him to take the drug an hour before meals. Food in the GI tract may reduce absorption.

*Note:* Captopril is currently under study as an option for treating mild hypertension. Recent research suggests that it's less likely to cause adverse reactions than originally believed.

# STEP 4

## PREPARING YOUR PATIENT FOR STEP 4 THERAPY

Because Step 4 drugs are highly potent, take special care when preparing a patient for Step 4 therapy. First, review the basics of hypertension control. Then, stress that the potency of the drug he's about to take makes being conscientious more important than ever. Go over the manufacturer's drug information insert with him. Emphasize the need to continue all prescribed medications and keep his follow-up appointments. Emphasize that the doctor can reduce or eliminate possible adverse reactions by adjusting the drug's dosage or substituting another drug.

**Guanethidine sulfate.** If your patient begins taking this drug, warn him that he's likely to feel dizzy when he first stands up, especially when he gets out of bed in the morning. Standing for long periods, exercising heavily, or drinking alcohol may also cause dizziness, so he should avoid or minimize these activities. As with all of the antihypertensive drugs in stepped-care therapy, reporting adverse reactions to the doctor is important.

**Guanadrel sulfate.** Special considerations for the patient taking this relatively new drug are similar to those for guanethidine. For details about guanadrel, see the following page.

**Minoxidil.** Tell a patient taking this drug to watch out for fluid retention and instruct him to immediately report any sudden weight gain, breathing difficulty, or swelling in his hands or feet. Also, let him know that minoxidil sometimes causes facial and body hair to thicken or darken.

**Captopril.** As a rule, captopril is given with a diuretic. Your patient must take this drug an hour before meals; help him think of ways to remember to do so. If he becomes dehydrated, his blood pressure may drop suddenly and severely. If he's taking a diuretic, suggest that he drink more water when he's perspiring heavily. Advise him to notify the doctor if dizziness persists.

Explain that captopril sometimes causes complications that can become severe if not caught quickly. For example, to head off infection from neutropenia (a possible adverse reaction of the drug), he must notify the doctor of such symptoms as mouth sores, sore throat, or fever. Explain that you'll check him regularly for signs of proteinuria, another potential problem.

## COMPARING THERAPEUTIC EFFECTIVENESS

| DRUG | ROUTE | ONSET | DURATION |
|---|---|---|---|
| guanethidine sulfate | P.O. | 1 to 3 weeks | 1 to 3 weeks |
| minoxidil | P.O. | 30 minutes | 24 hours |
| captopril | P.O. | 1 hour | 6 to 12 hours |

## ANTICIPATING DRUG INTERACTIONS

Make sure you know all possible interactions before you administer any drugs to your patient, and warn him against taking any additional drugs without his doctor's approval. For a look at how two Step 4 drugs interact with other drugs, see the chart below. Consult the manufacturer's package insert for more details.

*Note:* Captopril causes no significant interactions.

| DRUG | ▶TAKEN WITH | ▶CAUSES THIS INTERACTION |
|---|---|---|
| guanethidine sulfate | alcohol | Orthostatic hypotension and drowsiness |
| | amphetamines | Decreased antihypertensive effect |
| | cyclic antidepressants | Decreased antihypertensive effect |
| | ephedrine | Decreased antihypertensive effect |
| | levarterenol (norepinephrine) | Increased antihypertensive effect; may cause cardiac dysrhythmias |
| | methylphenidate | Decreased antihypertensive effect |
| | MAO inhibitors | Decreased antihypertensive effect |
| | minoxidil | Severe orthostatic hypotension |
| | phenothiazines (especially chlorpromazine) | Decreased antihypertensive effect |
| minoxidil | guanethidine sulfate | Severe orthostatic hypotension |

## SCREENING FOR URINE PROTEIN

Rita Reilly, age 45, is taking captopril along with hydrochlorothiazide (HydroDIURIL) to control her hypertension. One in every hundred patients receiving captopril develops proteinuria, although the exact relationship between the drug and proteinuria is unclear. Because proteinuria may indicate kidney damage, screen your patient for this condition by monitoring her urine protein level at least monthly—and daily if the level rises.

For accurate results, test a clean-catch urine specimen—preferably one collected first thing in the morning when the urine is highly concentrated and yields the most reliable information. Then, immerse a reagent strip into the specimen for 1 second.

Remove the strip from the

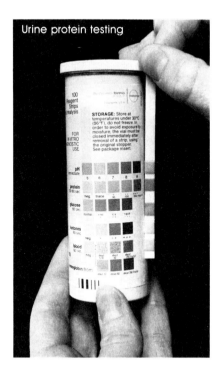

Urine protein testing

specimen, and tap it against the specimen container to shake off the excess urine. Compare the test-block color with the bottle's color chart, as shown at left.

Test results correspond to mg/dl of protein (usually albumin, since the reagent strips are most sensitive to albumin). Document your findings, using the guidelines in the box below.

> 0 to 5 mg/dl: Negative
> 5 to 20 mg/dl: Trace
> 30 mg/dl: 1+
> 100 mg/dl: 2+
> 300 mg/dl: 3+
> 1,000 mg/dl: 4+

If the test shows proteinuria in excess of 100 mg/dl, or if a less severe protein elevation persists, let the doctor know. He'll reevaluate captopril therapy.

## DRUG UPDATE

### GUANADREL SULFATE: HOW IT STACKS UP WITH GUANETHIDINE SULFATE

Like its close relative guanethidine sulfate, guanadrel sulfate (Hylorel*) lowers blood pressure by inhibiting norepinephrine release and depleting norepinephrine stores in peripheral nerve endings. Although indications, contraindications, and dosage are similar for these two drugs, guanadrel has some important distinctions. For example, it takes effect far more quickly than gua-

nethidine: within 4 to 6 hours following a single oral dose, compared to a week or longer for guanethidine. In addition, guanadrel's effects cease within 10 to 14 hours; guanethidine's effects may linger for a week or more.

Both drugs can cause such adverse reactions as dizziness, orthostatic hypotension, sexual dysfunction, and diarrhea. But perhaps because its duration of action is shorter, guanadrel is less likely to cause severe morning orthostatic hypotension or diarrhea.

Because both of these drugs cause unpleasant adverse reactions, the doctor may try to avoid prescribing either of them. But if treatment with one drug is indicated, guanadrel may have the edge.

When prescribing guanadrel, the doctor will also order a diuretic, because guanadrel causes water retention. For this reason, guanadrel is contraindicated for patients with congestive heart failure and other disorders related to fluid retention.

*Not available in Canada

# CALCIUM CHANNEL BLOCKERS

## CALCIUM CHANNEL BLOCKERS: A PROMISING ALTERNATIVE

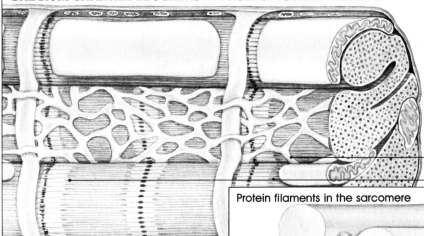

### Cross section of a muscle fiber

Calcium is stored in a muscle fiber's sarcoplasmic reticulum (see illustration at left). When muscle cells depolarize, they release calcium. Calcium permits binding between two protein filaments called actin and myosin, causing the fiber's sarcomeres to shorten and the fiber to contract.

The illustration below is a conceptual representation of the cross-bridges that form when actin and myosin bind together.

Sarcoplasmic reticulum

Sarcomere

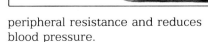

### Protein filaments in the sarcomere

Actin

Myosin

Cross-bridge

Sometime soon, you may find yourself caring for a hypertensive patient who's being treated with one of these calcium channel blockers: verapamil, nifedipine, or diltiazem. All three drugs are currently approved to treat severe angina; verapamil is also prescribed to treat dysrhythmias. These drugs may soon become options for treating hypertension, too. When you consider calcium's effects in the body, you can understand why.

**Calcium's role.** Calcium plays a part in almost every chemical process in the body. Most importantly, it:
• helps transmit electrical impulses in the heart
• enhances myocardial contractility
• causes smooth-muscle contraction in both peripheral and coronary arteries
• helps cells store and use energy.

All calcium channel blockers inhibit the movement of calcium into cells. By inhibiting calcium flow into arterial smooth-muscle cells, calcium blockers allow the vessels to relax and dilate. Arterial dilation, in turn, lowers peripheral resistance and reduces blood pressure.

**How calcium blockers differ.** All calcium blockers have both cardiac and vascular effects. But the strength of these effects varies among the drugs. Verapamil, for example, inhibits cardiac conduction and contractility, while nifedipine has little effect on either. Although diltiazem has some effect on conduction and contractility, its effect is less powerful than verapamil's.

How else do these drugs compare? Consider the following points:
• Nifedipine is the most powerful vasodilator of the three. Its effects are similar to those of hydralazine hydrochloride, a Step 3 vasodilator. But unlike hydralazine, nifedipine also reduces coronary artery resistance, providing better blood flow in the coronary arteries. As a result, it's especially promising for treating hypertensive patients who also have coronary artery disease.
• Verapamil, also a potent vasodilator, acts primarily on peripheral vessels. Like nifedipine, it also dilates coronary arteries.
• Diltiazem acts primarily on coronary arteries and has not been studied extensively as an antihypertensive drug. Of the three calcium channel blockers, it may prove to be the least suitable for hypertension management.

For a more detailed look at these three drugs, see the following chart.

*Note:* Calcium channel blockers are also called calcium antagonists and slow-channel blockers. The term *slow channel* refers to the relatively slow flow of calcium into cells during depolarization.

# LEARNING ABOUT CALCIUM CHANNEL BLOCKERS

| NIFEDIPINE |
| Procardia* |

## Indications
Angina from coronary artery spasm, chronic stable angina. Its use in hypertension management is under investigation.

## Dosage
Starting dosage: 10 mg P.O. or 10 mg sublingually, t.i.d.; gradually increase to maintenance dosage of 30 to 120 mg/day (30 to 60 mg daily for mild to moderate hypertension) in three to six divided doses. Maximum dosage: 120 mg/day.

## Possible adverse reactions
Dizziness, light-headedness, facial flushing, peripheral edema, nervousness, mood changes, palpitations, dyspnea, coughing, nasal congestion, wheezing, sore throat, headache, constipation

## Special considerations
• Give cautiously during pregnancy.
• To administer nifedipine sublingually (for example, to treat hypertensive crisis), puncture the capsule with a needle, withdraw the drug, and instill the drug under the patient's tongue.
• Monitor blood pressure carefully during initial therapy, especially in patients taking other antihypertensive drugs; nifedipine may also cause hypotension.
• When giving nifedipine with a beta blocker, watch for increased peripheral edema from vasodilation and angina (a less likely complication) from reflex tachycardia.

| VERAPAMIL |
| Calan*, Isoptin* |

## Indications
Angina pectoris. Its use in hypertension management is under investigation.

## Dosage
Starting dosage: from 80 (the usual starting dose) up to 160 mg P.O. t.i.d.; gradually increase to maintenance dosage of 240 to 480 mg/day in divided doses. Dosages as high as 720 mg/day may be given.

## Possible adverse reactions
Headache, hypotension, atrioventricular (AV) block, constipation, vertigo, nervousness, hepatotoxicity

## Special considerations
• Contraindicated in severe hypotension or cardiogenic shock; second- or third-degree AV block; sick sinus syndrome (except in patients with a pacemaker); and severe congestive heart failure.
• Use with extreme caution in combination with a beta blocker; the drug combination may contribute to heart failure.
• Use cautiously in patients with hepatic failure and renal failure; these conditions may prolong the effects of verapamil.
• Use cautiously in pregnancy. Advise lactating women to discontinue nursing during verapamil therapy.
• Use cautiously in patients taking protein-bound drugs (such as warfarin) and oral hypoglycemics.
• Watch for signs of second- or third-degree AV block, bradycardia, and asystole, especially in patients with sick sinus syndrome.
• If ordered, give verapamil with oral antihypertensive drugs. Monitor the patient for hypotension.
• Monitor serum digoxin levels during the first week of verapamil therapy—verapamil can increase serum digoxin levels.

• Use caution when giving verapamil with quinidine or propranolol hydrochloride. Either combination may cause hypotension.
• If your patient's receiving calcium supplements, closely monitor him for elevated serum calcium levels and check his pulse for irregularities.

| DILTIAZEM |
| Cardizem* |

## Indications
Angina pectoris from coronary artery spasm, chronic stable angina. Its use in hypertension management is under investigation.

## Dosage
Starting dosage: 30 mg q.i.d.; gradually increase to maintenance dosage of 240 mg/day in divided doses.

## Possible adverse reactions
Headache, hypotension, flushing, AV block, swelling, edema, nausea, dizziness, drug rash, constipation

## Special considerations
• Contraindicated in sick sinus syndrome (except in patients with a pacemaker); second- or third-degree AV block; and hypotension.
• Use cautiously with beta blockers or digitalis; may prolong conduction through the AV node.
• Use cautiously during pregnancy.
• Use cautiously in nursing women and in patients with impaired renal or hepatic function.
• Watch for occasional symptomatic hypotension.

*Not available in Canada

# DEALING WITH SPECIAL PROBLEMS

So far, we've focused on uncomplicated primary hypertension in otherwise healthy adults. Now, let's consider the hypertensive patient whose condition is complicated by a special problem.

For instance, if your patient experiences hypertensive crisis, can you promptly recognize this life-threatening complication—and correctly administer the potent antihypertensive drugs the doctor will order? Read the next few pages for guidelines.

Unless you're an ob/gyn nurse, you may have little experience with pregnancy-induced hypertension (also called preeclampsia). That's why we've provided detailed information about this dangerous condition that threatens both mother and child.

We've also provided details on pheochromocytoma and renovascular hypertension. And we discuss hemorrhagic stroke, a possible complication of either primary or secondary hypertension.

Finally, you'll see how to adapt all you've learned about hypertension management for pediatric and geriatric patients.

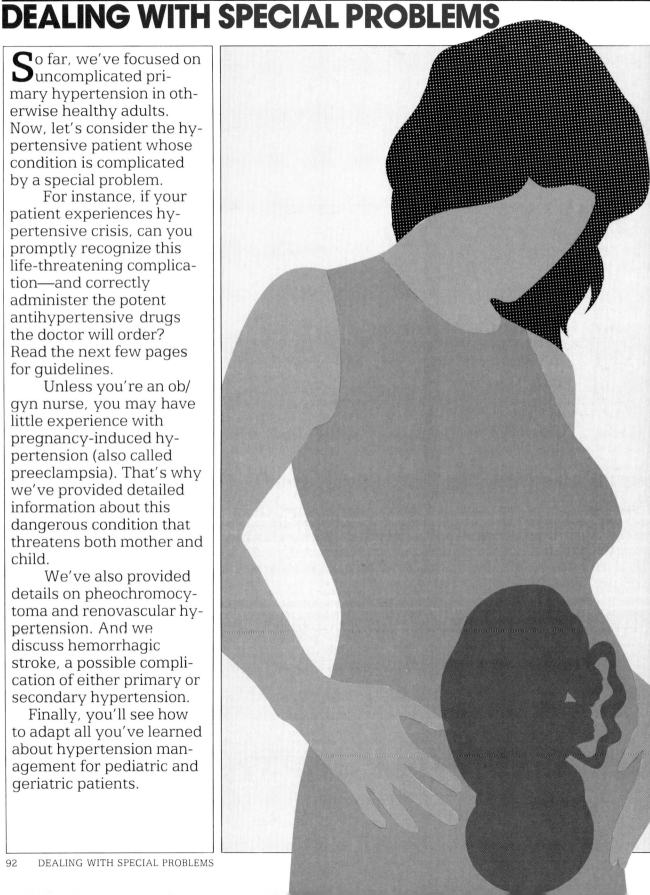

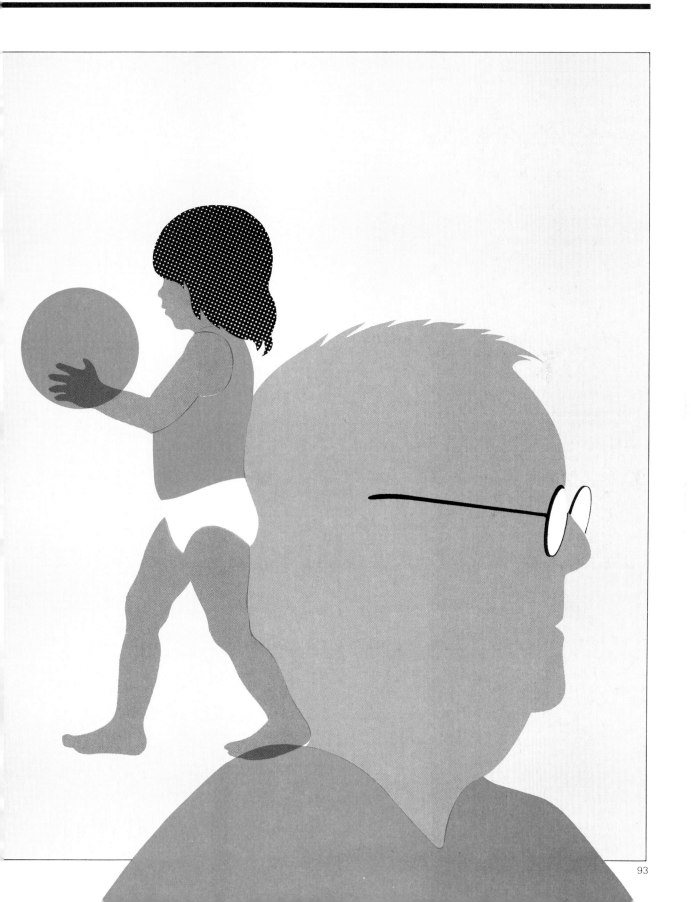

# HYPERTENSIVE CRISIS

### HYPERTENSIVE CRISIS: A CASE IN POINT

Neil Richards, a 47-year-old executive, is rushed to the emergency department after developing a severe headache and blurred vision at work. When he arrives, his blood pressure measurement is 260/170 mm Hg. He seems agitated and confused and is having difficulty breathing. His company's nurse, who accompanied him to the hospital, supplies you with the following history.

Six months ago, Mr. Richards found out that he's hypertensive. Since then, he's been controlling the problem with diet and medication. However, he's not always as careful about taking his medications as he should be. In fact, he recently told the company nurse that he sometimes forgets to take them when he's feeling particularly well. Despite her efforts to encourage his compliance, she suspects that he's neglected his medication during the past week.

With this background, you can probably anticipate the doctor's diagnosis—hypertensive crisis. Although a patient like Mr. Richards may be transferred to the intensive care unit, you're responsible for recognizing the problem and providing appropriate interim care. Make sure you can meet the challenge by reading the following pages.

### WHAT CAUSES CRISIS?

The sudden, extreme, and life-threatening blood pressure elevation known as hypertensive crisis may be caused by any number of conditions. Primary hypertension can lead to crisis if the condition isn't treated properly and an acute blood pressure increase occurs; or if an acute blood pressure increase is accompanied by a complication such as an acute dissecting aortic aneurysm, a leaking abdominal aortic aneurysm, or an intracranial hemorrhage.

Secondary hypertension can also cause hypertensive crisis if the primary condition—for example, pheochromocytoma, acute or chronic glomerulonephritis, renovascular hypertension, or pregnancy-induced hypertension (PIH)—becomes more severe.

Antihypertensive drug withdrawal can cause crisis, too. Consider Mr. Richards, for example. You suspect that he's neglected to take his antihypertensive drugs for the past week or so. If you're correct, his noncompliance is the most likely cause of crisis.

Interactions between foods and drugs are another possible cause of hypertensive crisis. If your patient's taking a monoamine oxidase (MAO) inhibitor, such as pargyline hydrochloride or phenelzine sulfate (Nardil), he's at risk of crisis if he eats or drinks anything containing tyramine—for example, avocados, Chianti wine, imported beer, chicken livers, chocolate, meats prepared with tenderizers, caviar, pickled herring, sausage meats, aged or processed cheese, or yeast extract.

Similarly, some drug interactions can trigger hypertensive crisis; for example, an interaction between guanethidine sulfate and cyclic antidepressants.

### RECOGNIZING HYPERTENSIVE CRISIS

How do you know whether your patient's in hypertensive crisis? Surprisingly, his blood pressure reading isn't the most valuable indicator. What's important is whether his life is in immediate danger from cerebral, cardiovascular, or renal compromise. In other words, if your hypertensive patient's diastolic pressure is 140 but he's resting comfortably, then he's *not* in crisis. On the other hand, you *should* suspect crisis if your previously diagnosed hypertensive patient has some or all of the signs and symptoms listed below—even if his diastolic pressure is only moderately high.

Signs and symptoms that may accompany hypertensive crisis include:
• headache
• nausea and vomiting
• blurred vision
• drowsiness
• confusion
• limb numbness or tingling
• convulsions
• coma
• azotemia
• chest pain
• oliguria
• hemorrhagic exudates and papilledema on funduscopy
• shortness of breath.

*Important:* Signs and symptoms of hypertensive crisis may mimic those of other life-threatening conditions, such as CVA. Take into consideration the entire clinical picture—including the patient's history—before making a judgment. For guidelines on distinguishing CVA from hypertensive crisis, see the box on the following page.

## HOW CRISIS AFFECTS TARGET ORGANS

Four target organs are most severely affected by acute high blood pressure—the brain, eyes, heart, and kidney. Let's take a close look at the effects on each organ.

**The brain.** Although no one knows exactly how crisis affects the brain, two theories offer possible explanations. One is that crisis causes severe vasoconstriction. Vasoconstriction, in turn, may lead to cerebral ischemia and tissue damage.

The other possibility is that disturbances in the blood-brain barrier associated with acute hypertension allow fluid to accumulate in brain tissue. As edema builds, your patient shows signs and symptoms of hypertensive encephalopathy: severe headache, agitation or irritability, nausea and vomiting, blurred vision, drowsiness, confusion, numbness or tingling in arms or legs, convulsions, and coma.

**The eye.** You'll see the effects of severe vasoconstriction when you examine your patient's retinal arteries. During a funduscopic exam, the retinal arteries may appear thready and one-third to one-fourth their normal size. Or, you may not be able to see them at all. If your patient suffered accelerated or malignant hypertension before the crisis occurred, you may also see grade III or IV retinopathy (see pages 34 and 35 for details).

**The heart.** During hypertensive crisis, high blood pressure increases heart wall stress. As pressure builds, blood flow to the heart's subendocardial layer decreases. As the wall becomes ischemic, the left ventricle's compliance decreases, raising left ventricular end-diastolic pressure (filling pressure). Rising pressure and ischemia cause the heart to

## HYPERTENSIVE CRISIS OR CVA?

Because signs and symptoms are similar, distinguishing hypertensive crisis from CVA isn't easy. But trying to do so is important, because the diagnosis affects the choice of treatment. If your patient's in hypertensive crisis, the doctor will lower blood pressure rapidly. But if the patient's suffered a CVA, the doctor will lower blood pressure more gradually.

Suspect CVA if your patient:
• shows focal or lateralizing neurologic signs, rather than generalized ones.
• develops neurologic deficits suddenly, rather than progressively.

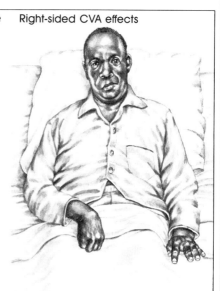
Right-sided CVA effects

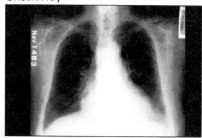
Chest X-ray

Left ventricular hypertrophy, shown in the X-ray above, contributes to heart failure during hypertensive crisis.

The X-ray at upper right shows constriction of both renal arteries (see arrows). The right renal artery is more constricted than the left.

At right, a CT scan reveals left frontal hemorrhage (the white area) and surrounding edema (the black area).

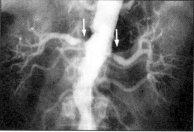
Renal arteriogram

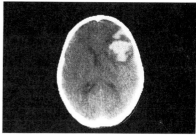
CT scan: Head

pump less efficiently. Then, as the heart begins to fail, blood backs up into the lungs, causing pulmonary edema. (Remember, the left ventricle may already be compromised by hypertrophy, a common complication of sustained hypertension.) Consequently, the hypertensive crisis patient may suffer acute shortness of breath.

**The kidney.** Just as hypertensive crisis causes severe cerebral vasoconstriction, crisis may cause severe vasoconstriction of the kidney's arterioles. Impaired renal circulation causes proteinuria, microscopic hematuria, and renal insufficiency leading to renal failure.

*Note*: Hypertensive crisis may also cause hemolytic anemia resulting from red blood cell damage secondary to vasoconstriction.

# HYPERTENSIVE CRISIS

## MAINTAINING SECONDARY I.V. LINES: THREE OPTIONS

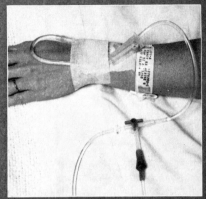

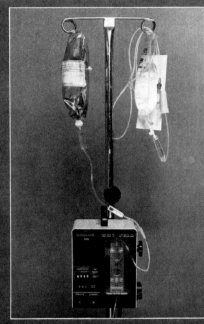

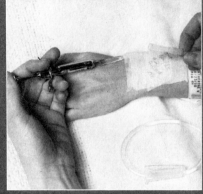

When your patient's in hypertensive crisis, the drugs she's receiving to lower her dangerously high blood pressure are so potent that her blood pressure could plummet to hypotensive levels in just a few minutes. As a result, you may need to discontinue drug therapy quickly while maintaining the I.V. line's patency. Here are three ways to do this.

Piggyback a secondary I.V. line using a stopcock, as shown above, so you can easily turn off the line that's infusing the drug. Turn the stopcock to the proper position so the secondary line remains open. In this case, you'd turn the stopcock clockwise.

Discontinue the drug and convert the I.V. to a heparin lock (see photo above). *Note:* Keep heparin flush solution, normal saline solution, and an I.V. cap by the patient's bedside so you can convert the line quickly.

Keep a secondary I.V. bag (usually containing dextrose 5% in water) handy, as shown at left. If you need to stop the drug, disconnect the drug line and connect the secondary I.V. line.

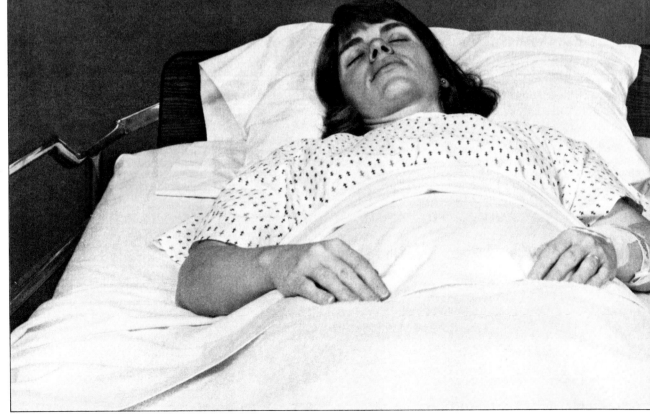

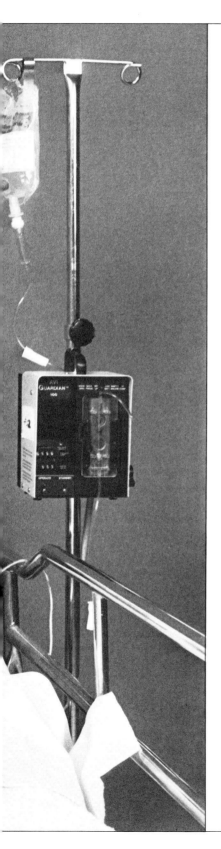

## INTERVENTION: YOUR ROLE

Your patient's in hypertensive crisis. What should you do? Of course, your actions depend on the patient's status, the presence of any complications (such as pulmonary edema), and doctor's orders. But in general, follow these guidelines:

• Establish an I.V. setup that will permit you to quickly discontinue the antihypertensive drug, if necessary, without sacrificing the line's patency. For a look at several suitable setups, see the photos at left.

• Give antihypertensive drugs, as ordered (see the chart on pages 98 and 99). To ensure accurate drug dosage, use an infusion pump.

• If your patient doesn't have an arterial line in place, document his blood pressure at least every 2 minutes (or as ordered) during initial drug therapy; less frequently (but regularly) as his condition stabilizes. Or, use an automatic blood pressure device, like the Dinamap shown on page 41. Notify the doctor immediately if the patient becomes hypotensive and adjust drug therapy as ordered.

• Monitor and record the patient's pulse rate, respiratory status, and fluid intake and output. Record these readings on a flowchart, if used.

• If ordered, gather equipment for an arterial line.

• Document any changes in the patient's physical or mental status, all medications administered, and laboratory test results.

## LOWERING BLOOD PRESSURE: THE TOP PRIORITY

Your first priority when treating the patient in hypertensive crisis is to lower his blood pressure. How? By administering antihypertensive drugs parenterally, as the doctor orders.

On the next two pages, we've provided a chart detailing the antihypertensive drugs commonly ordered to treat hypertensive crisis. Study this chart carefully. Remember, these drugs are so potent that, if administered incorrectly, they may cause hypotension and trigger a heart attack or stroke.

**A typical protocol.** Even though your patient's in crisis, the doctor will begin treatment with a low drug dose. Then, he'll evaluate the patient's response before proceeding. This cautious approach lessens the risk of extreme vasodilation and dangerous hypotension.

Unless the patient responds dramatically, the doctor then gradually increases the infusion rate until the patient's blood pressure starts dropping. Then, he'll order a maintenance infusion rate. Once blood pressure stabilizes at the desired level (this may take days), the transition from I.V. to oral medication begins.

**Precautions.** Make sure that every medication change is preceded and followed by a blood pressure reading. Watch closely for hypotension and for signs of heart failure, such as tachycardia, tachypnea, dyspnea, pulmonary rales, $S_3$ sounds, neck vein distention, and edema.

# HYPERTENSIVE CRISIS

## HYPERTENSIVE CRISIS: A GUIDE TO DRUGS

To treat hypertensive crisis, the doctor will order an I.V. antihypertensive drug—stat. All of the drugs listed in the following chart combat hypertensive crisis by lowering blood pressure quickly. Because they're so powerful, you must take special care whenever giving these drugs. No matter which one the doctor orders, keep these guidelines in mind:
• Give I.V. infusions with an infusion pump, for dosage accuracy.
• Constantly monitor the patient's condition. Take his blood pressure and other vital signs frequently during the drug infusion. Watch for signs of hypotension.
• Prepare him for transfer to the intensive care unit, if ordered, for continuous cardiac and hemodynamic monitoring.

### DIAZOXIDE (Hyperstat)

Similar in chemical composition to thiazide diuretics, yet paradoxically causes sodium and water retention. Lowers blood pressure by dilating peripheral arterioles.

**Dosage**
Administer 300 mg (or 5 mg/kg body weight) I.V. bolus into a peripheral vein within 30 seconds; repeat at intervals of 4 to 24 hours, as necessary. Or, give 1 to 3 mg/kg I.V. bolus to maximum of 150 mg at intervals of 5 to 15 minutes. Or, give by infusion at a rate of 15 mg/minute over 20 to 30 minutes.
*Note:* A series of low-dose injections lowers the risk of stroke or myocardial infarction (MI) by lowering blood pressure more gradually.

**Onset and duration**
*Onset:* 3 to 5 minutes
*Duration:* 2 to 18 hours

**Adverse reactions**
Sodium and water retention, hyperglycemia, headache, vomiting

**Nursing considerations**
• Contraindicated in patients with aortic dissection.
• Use cautiously in patients with coronary insufficiency; vasodilation, reflex tachycardia, increased cardiac output, and negative inotropism (all characteristic drug effects) may lead to MI if heart is already compromised.
• Use cautiously in cerebrovascular insufficiency (drug may precipitate stroke) and in patients with diabetes (drug may cause significant temporary hyperglycemia).
• Check blood pressure every 3 to 5 minutes for the first 30 minutes.
• Watch the I.V. insertion site for signs of extravasation, since this drug is very irritating to the tissues.
• Monitor fluid intake and output. Begin diuretic therapy within 24 to 48 hours, as ordered; diazoxide causes fluid retention.
• Monitor the patient for ischemic changes, including angina and dysrhythmias.
• For patients receiving multiple injections, monitor serum glucose levels daily. Previously controlled diabetic patients may need more insulin than usual.
*Caution:* Patients receiving anticoagulants may need dosage reductions, because diazoxide displaces coumarin from serum albumin.
• Replace the I.V. drug with an oral antihypertensive drug as soon as possible.

### HYDRALAZINE HYDROCHLORIDE (Apresoline)

Lowers blood pressure by dilating peripheral arterioles; also increases renal blood flow. Is not consistently effective in treating hypertensive encephalopathy.

**Dosage**
*For intermittent injection,* give 20 to 40 mg diluted to 20 ml, administered no faster than 1 ml/minute, until blood pressure drops to desired level.
*For continuous infusion,* give 50 to 100 mg/liter, and titrate according to blood pressure response. (The doctor may order a continuous infusion to treat eclampsia.)

**Onset and duration**
*Onset:* 10 to 15 minutes
*Duration:* 3 to 8 hours

**Adverse reactions**
Headache, tachycardia, angina, water retention, vomiting, diarrhea

**Nursing considerations**
• Contraindicated for patients with acute coronary insufficiency and for patients with dissecting aneurysm.
• Use cautiously if patient is receiving other antihypertensive medication, especially diazoxide.
• Check blood pressure and pulse rate every 3 to 5 minutes.
• Monitor the patient for tachycardia, ischemic changes, and dysrhythmias.
• Observe for nausea and vomiting.
• Replace I.V. drug with an oral antihypertensive drug as soon as possible.

### NITROPRUSSIDE SODIUM (Nipride)

Relaxes both arteriolar and venular smooth muscle. Potent and effective, nitroprusside is the drug of choice for most patients in hypertensive crisis.

**Dosage**
Dissolve 50 mg of nitroprusside in 2 to 3 ml of dextrose 5% in water; then add to 250 ml of dextrose 5% in water. Administer solution only by infusion pump or microdrip regulator. Reconstituted solution is stable for 24 hours if protected from light.
*Average dose:* 3 mcg/kg/minute
*Dosage range:* 0.5 to 10 mcg/kg/minute

## Onset and duration

*Onset:* Within seconds
*Duration:* 1 to 5 minutes

## Adverse reactions

Headache, dizziness, diaphoresis, muscle twitching, vomiting, abdominal or chest pain, palpitations. *Note:* Nitroprusside rarely causes adverse reactions except in overdose or when given too rapidly. Side effects associated with overly rapid administration are nausea, vomiting, muscle twitching, drowsiness, and restlessness.

## Nursing considerations

• Contraindicated when continuous hemodynamic monitoring isn't available.
• Mark the drug container with the time and date the solution was prepared.
• If required by hospital policy, cover the tubing and/or container with aluminum foil or another opaque wrapping, to protect the solution from light. (Although standard practice in the past, protecting nitroprusside from light is not now considered mandatory by all authorities.)
• Discard darkly tinted solution (fresh solution has a slightly brown tint).
• Monitor blood pressure continuously, and watch for signs of hypotension.
• Watch for these signs and symptoms of thiocyanate accumulation: tinnitus, blurred vision, delirium, acidosis, and hypoxia.
   *Caution:* In long-term use, nitroprusside may cause cyanide poisoning.
• Monitor the I.V. insertion site for signs of extravasation.

---

### PHENTOLAMINE HYDROCHLORIDE, PHENTOLAMINE METHANESULFONATE (Regitine*)

Acts as an alpha blocker; causes vasodilation. Is especially useful to treat hypertensive crisis associated with excess catecholamines; for example, crisis from pheochromocytoma, food interactions with monoamine oxidase (MAO) inhibitors, and abrupt clonidine hydrochloride withdrawal.

## Dosage

Give 5 to 20 mg I.V. bolus, followed by 0.2 to 5 mg/minute I.V. infusion or 2.5 to 5 mg I.V. every 5 minutes until patient responds; then, bolus every 2 to 4 hours.

## Onset and duration

*Onset:* Within seconds
*Duration:* Less than 5 minutes

## Adverse reactions

Dizziness, tachycardia, cardiac dysrhythmias, vomiting, diarrhea, nasal congestion

## Nursing considerations

• Contraindicated in patients with angina, coronary artery disease, and a history of myocardial infarction.
• Use cautiously in patients with gastritis or peptic ulcer and in those receiving other antihypertensive drugs.
• If ordered, give norepinephrine (Levophed) to reverse a severe blood pressure drop.
• Check blood pressure and heart rate frequently until the patient's condition is stable.
• Monitor patient for dysrhythmias and tachycardia.

---

### TRIMETHAPHAN CAMSYLATE (Arfonad)

Blocks sympathetic and parasympathetic nerve impulses. May be ordered if the patient doesn't respond to nitroprusside.

## Dosage

Administer 1,000 mg/liter continuous I.V. infusion at 0.5 to 4 mg/minute, to a maximum dosage of 15 mg/minute. Titrate dosage to blood pressure response.

## Onset and duration

*Onset:* 1 to 2 minutes
*Duration:* 5 minutes

## Adverse reactions

Urinary retention, weakness, tachycardia, vomiting, dry mouth, paralytic ileus, dilated pupils

## Nursing considerations

• Contraindicated in patients with anemia or respiratory insufficiency.
• Use cautiously in patients with glaucoma; arteriosclerosis; cardiac, renal, or hepatic disease; degenerative central nervous system disorders; Addison's disease; lower urinary tract obstruction; or diabetes.
• Use cautiously in patients taking glucocorticoids or antihypertensive drugs.
• Maximize drug's effect by raising the head of the bed 4" to 6" (10 to 15 cm). This encourages blood to pool in the lower extremities, reducing venous return.
• Give with a diuretic, if ordered.
• Monitor fluid intake and output. If ordered, insert an indwelling Foley catheter, to relieve urinary retention.
• Expect the patient's pupils to dilate; keep this in mind when doing a neurologic assessment.
• Observe for refractory blood pressure changes after 48 hours of drug therapy.

# P.I.H.

## HYPERTENSION AND PREGNANCY

Granted, treating any patient with hypertension is a complex job with many special considerations. But, treating a *pregnant* patient with hypertension is even more complicated. Obviously, you and the doctor want to lower her blood pressure. The challenge is to do so without jeopardizing the fetus, since lowering blood pressure may decrease the blood supply to the placenta and deprive the fetus of oxygen. On the following pages, we'll discuss this and other problems associated with hypertension in pregnancy.

Your patient may have been hypertensive before she became pregnant. (We'll discuss chronic hypertension and pregnancy on page 105.) Or, she may have developed hypertension as a result of her pregnancy. The latter condition is called *pregnancy-induced hypertension* (PIH), formerly known as toxemia of pregnancy.

PIH occurs most often in primigravidas younger than age 20 or older than age 35. Its first stage (preeclampsia) usually develops after the 20th week of gestation. In addition to the high blood pressure that's characteristic of preeclampsia, the patient's symptoms often include proteinuria and edema.

If her condition isn't treated (or isn't treated properly), it can progress to eclampsia—the later, more dangerous stage of PIH. Eclampsia, characterized by seizures and possibly coma, threatens both mother and fetus. Read on to find out more about how PIH develops—and how you can intervene.

## NORMAL PREGNANCY: A REVIEW

Before you read about the pathophysiology of PIH, let's review the physiologic changes that normally occur during pregnancy. See the following page for illustrations of a fully developed fetus and placenta.

**Increased blood volume.** During pregnancy, maternal blood volume increases anywhere from 30% to 50%. By increasing blood volume, the body meets the increased demand for blood from both the fetus and the mother. This increase in blood volume also helps minimize the effects of decreased venous circulation that occur during maternal position changes.

**Decreased blood pressure.** In response to increased blood volume, heart rate quickens and stroke volume rises. As a result, cardiac output (CO) increases. Normally, increased CO causes blood pressure to rise if peripheral vascular resistance (PVR) remains constant. (BP = CO x PVR.) But during pregnancy, arteriolar dilation occurs, probably from increased progesterone levels, and peripheral resistance drops. Consequently, diastolic blood pressure drops about

20 mm Hg during the first and second trimesters. During the third trimester, blood pressure returns to the patient's normal (prepregnancy) level.

**Increased renin-angiotensin-aldosterone production.** During pregnancy, the activity of the renin-angiotensin-aldosterone system is accelerated and plasma levels of renin and angiotensin II rise. This probably is from increased estrogen production during pregnancy. However, the pregnant woman normally develops resistance to the pressor effect of angiotensin II, preventing an increase in blood pressure.

The increased aldosterone level, also produced by the renin-angiotensin-aldosterone cycle, encourages sodium reabsorption and water retention. This increases total body water and contributes to increased plasma volume.

**Increased glomerular filtration.** Increased blood volume, as well as arteriolar dilation, causes renal blood flow to increase by as much as 50% during pregnancy. Consequently, both the glomerular filtration rate and urine output increase.

## UNDERSTANDING P.I.H.

What causes PIH? At present, no one really knows. However, a link seems to exist between PIH and the number of chorionic villi (the fingerlike projections that form the placental tree) present. Women who develop a high number of chorionic villi—for example, during a first pregnancy or when carrying more than one fetus—are predisposed to PIH.

For reasons that remain unclear, women who develop PIH experience vasospasms, or arteriolar constriction. Arteriolar constriction, of course, increases peripheral resistance. As a result, the woman's systemic blood pressure rises.

How does hypertension affect the woman and her pregnancy? Read what follows for details.

**The effects of P.I.H.**

*Angiotensin II sensitivity.* During pregnancy, a woman normally produces high amounts of angiotensin II, yet becomes more resistant to its effects. In contrast, a woman with PIH produces *less* angiotensin II, yet becomes ex-

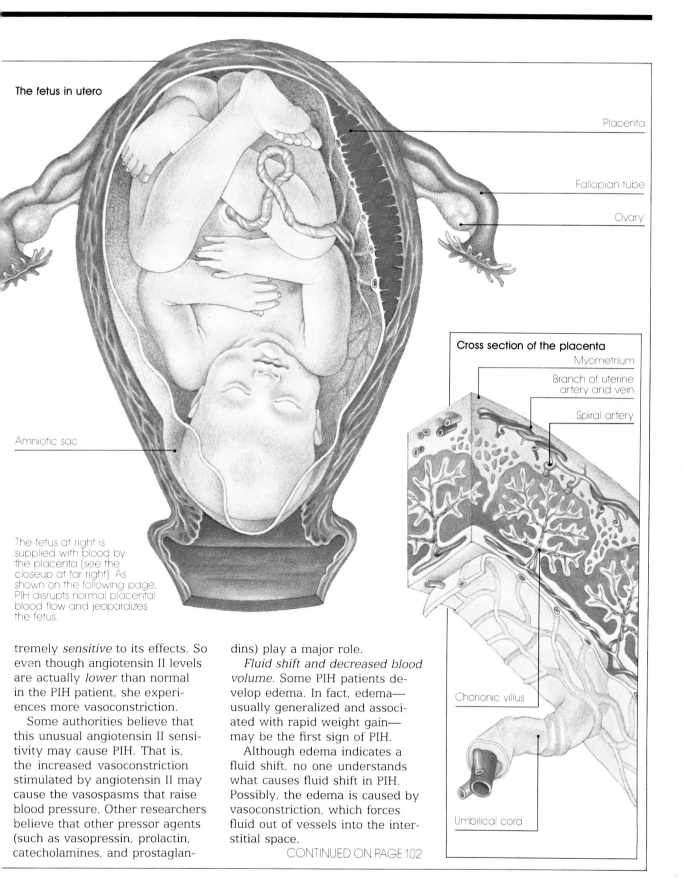

The fetus in utero

Placenta

Fallopian tube

Ovary

Amniotic sac

The fetus at right is supplied with blood by the placenta (see the closeup at far right). As shown on the following page, PIH disrupts normal placental blood flow and jeopardizes the fetus.

Cross section of the placenta

Myometrium

Branch of uterine artery and vein

Spiral artery

Chorionic villus

Umbilical cord

tremely *sensitive* to its effects. So even though angiotensin II levels are actually *lower* than normal in the PIH patient, she experiences more vasoconstriction.

Some authorities believe that this unusual angiotensin II sensitivity may cause PIH. That is, the increased vasoconstriction stimulated by angiotensin II may cause the vasospasms that raise blood pressure. Other researchers believe that other pressor agents (such as vasopressin, prolactin, catecholamines, and prostaglan-dins) play a major role.

*Fluid shift and decreased blood volume.* Some PIH patients develop edema. In fact, edema—usually generalized and associated with rapid weight gain—may be the first sign of PIH.

Although edema indicates a fluid shift, no one understands what causes fluid shift in PIH. Possibly, the edema is caused by vasoconstriction, which forces fluid out of vessels into the interstitial space.

CONTINUED ON PAGE 102

# P.I.H.

As PIH worsens, more fluid shifts to the interstitial space, circulating volume drops, and hematocrit rises. Normally, blood pressure drops when circulating volume decreases. But in PIH, vasospasm has reduced the size of the vascular bed. Because peripheral resistance is high, blood pressure doesn't drop.

*Decreased glomerular filtration.* Vasoconstriction decreases renal blood flow and the glomerular filtration rate. Glomeruli swell, becoming ischemic and partially occluded (a condition known as capillary endotheliosis). As capillary endotheliosis worsens, glomerular filtration decreases and the kidneys excrete more protein, causing proteinuria.

*Sodium and water retention.* The kidneys, sensing decreased blood volume, retain more sodium and water to increase blood volume.

*Disseminated intravascular coagulation (DIC).* As PIH worsens, DIC (abnormal clotting with thrombocytopenia) may develop. This condition may cause a seizure, profound generalized changes (tachycardia, restlessness, diaphoresis), and hemorrhage from any open wound. No one completely understands DIC or knows whether it's a cause or an effect of PIH.

*Decreased placental perfusion.* As pregnancy progresses, the placenta's spiral arteries normally lose vasomotor tone down to the radial artery. This permits generous blood flow to the placenta. But in PIH, the spiral arteries lose tone only down to the deciduomyometrial junction; the myometrial portions of the arteries retain muscular tone. As a result, the vasospasms characteristic of PIH affect the muscular portions of these arteries, causing constriction and decreased pla-

cental blood flow. The illustration above contrasts normal spiral arteries with those affected by PIH.

When placental blood flow is disrupted, the fetus can become undernourished and may be small for his gestational age. If blood flow is severely disrupted, the fetus may die.

*Increased intracellular sodium and decreased intracellular potassium.* Central nervous system (CNS) irritability develops as PIH worsens. Although the pathophysiology is unclear, increased sodium and decreased potassium in the cells may play a role. In some patients, these changes cause seizures.

**Spiral arteries: A closer look**

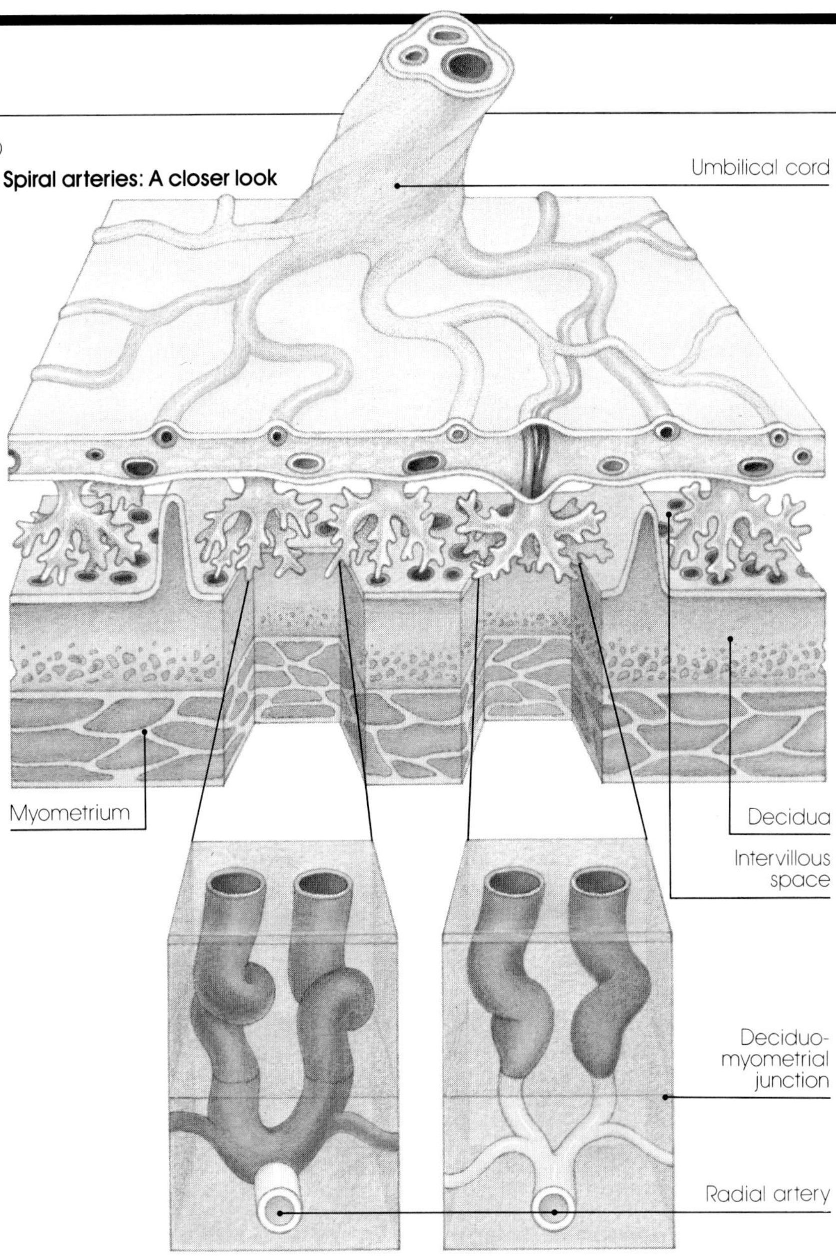

Umbilical cord

Myometrium

Decidua

Intervillous space

Deciduomyometrial junction

Radial artery

In a normal pregnancy, the spiral arteries lose muscular tone from the radial artery to the intervillous space, as shown in the closeup at left. This permits them to become passive, open channels.

In PIH, however, the spiral arteries lose tone only to the deciduomyometrial junction, as shown at right. As a result, they constrict in response to the vasospasms of PIH, restricting blood flow.

## CLASSIFYING PREECLAMPSIA

The severity of your patient's symptoms determines whether she has mild preeclampsia, severe preeclampsia, or eclampsia. Here's how to distinguish them.

**Mild preeclampsia**

• *hypertension:* blood pressure 140/90 mm Hg, or a systolic blood pressure 30 mm Hg higher than normal, or a diastolic blood pressure 15 mm Hg higher than normal. *Note:* When checking your patient for hypertension, take two blood pressure readings at least 6 hours apart. If possible, compare these readings with a baseline reading taken early in the patient's pregnancy (or prior to pregnancy).

• *edema:* sudden weight gain (more than 2 lb or 1 kg/week)

• *proteinuria:* excretion of 500 mg to 1 g or more in 24 hours; the presence of 2+ protein in a clean-catch, midstream urine specimen. (Bacteria, blood, or amniotic fluid in the urine can influence the amount of protein you detect.)

**Severe preeclampsia**

• *hypertension:* blood pressure 160/100 mm Hg or greater

• *edema:* drastic weight gain and edema of the face, hands, sacral area, lower extremities, and the abdominal wall

• *proteinuria:* excretion of 5 g or more in 24 hours; the presence of 3+ or 4+ protein in a clean-catch, midstream urine specimen.

**Signs of impending convulsion or seizure (eclampsia)**

• frontal headache, dizziness, blurred vision

• hyperreflexia of deep tendon reflexes

• epigastric pain

• impaired liver function

• thrombocytopenia

• oliguria (less than 400 ml/24 hours or less than 30 ml/hour).

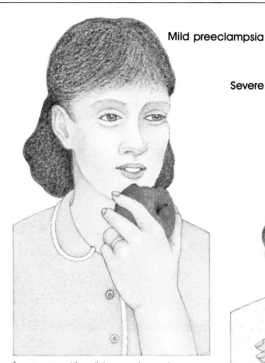

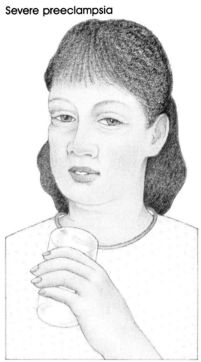

Mild preeclampsia

Severe preeclampsia

A woman with mild preeclampsia may show signs of edema, especially of the face and hands (see illustration above). As her condition becomes more severe, swelling worsens and her facial features appear coarse (as shown at right).

## PREDICTING P.I.H.

Can you anticipate PIH before clinical signs appear? In some cases, *yes*—with the help of one of the following tests. If the result of either of these tests is positive, teach the patient to report the signs and symptoms of PIH.

**The roll-over test.** Take the patient's blood pressure three times, under these circumstances: after she's been lying on her left side for 20 minutes; immediately after she turns onto her back; and 5 minutes later, while she's still lying on her back. If her diastolic blood pressure increases by 20 mm Hg according to either reading taken while she's on her back, the result is positive and she's at risk of developing PIH. *Note:* The roll-over test has a high false-positive rate (as high as 75%) and false-negative rate (about 30%).

**Angiotensin II infusion.** Since the roll-over test may be unreliable, the doctor may prefer to monitor the patient's blood pressure while she receives an infusion of angiotensin II. Because a pregnant woman with PIH is unusually sensitive to the pressor effects of angiotensin II, an angiotensin II infusion will provoke a more dramatic blood pressure increase if PIH is present than it would normally. Although this test is a more accurate predictor of PIH than the roll-over test, not all facilities are equipped to perform it. *Note:* Neither test is a substitute for ongoing assessment. Continue to monitor your patient's condition.

# P.I.H.

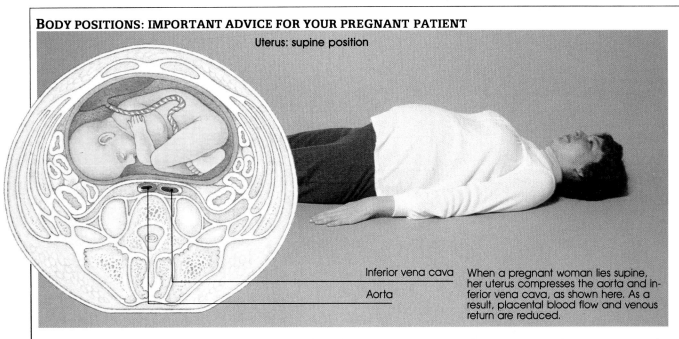

Uterus: supine position

Inferior vena cava

Aorta

When a pregnant woman lies supine, her uterus compresses the aorta and inferior vena cava, as shown here. As a result, placental blood flow and venous return are reduced.

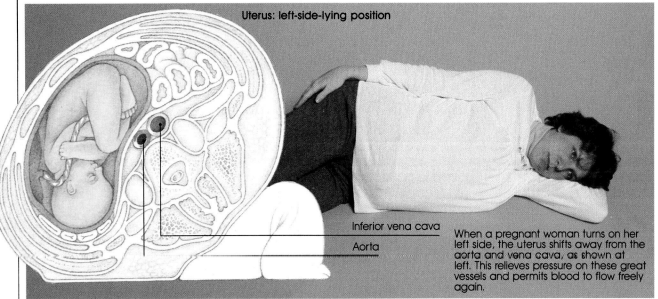

Uterus: left-side-lying position

Inferior vena cava

Aorta

When a pregnant woman turns on her left side, the uterus shifts away from the aorta and vena cava, as shown at left. This relieves pressure on these great vessels and permits blood to flow freely again.

Beth Miller, age 27, is 5 months pregnant. During a routine examination at the hospital clinic, you discover, for the second consecutive time, that her blood pressure is elevated (142/90 mm Hg). After the doctor examines Ms. Miller, he diagnoses her as mildly preeclamptic and tells her to rest for a few hours during the day on her left side.

Because you know the possible consequences of uncontrolled pregnancy-induced hypertension (PIH), take time to counsel Ms. Miller about the importance of following the doctor's orders carefully. Emphasize how sitting, standing, and lying positions affect her blood pressure—and what she can do to minimize the adverse effects of each position.

For guidelines on the advice to give a patient like Ms. Miller and the reasons behind your advice, read what follows. Make these guidelines a routine part of counseling for all your pregnant patients, especially those with PIH.
• *Don't sit or stand for long periods of time.* Whenever a person sits or stands, blood rushes into her legs and pools there. In a

pregnant woman, this pooling effect is compounded by pressure from the uterus on the abdominal and iliac veins. After about 10 minutes, hemoconcentration occurs as plasma moves out of blood vessels into the interstitial space. This process causes swelling in the legs and feet and a reduction in systemic blood volume, venous return, and cardiac output. To compensate for this reduction, the heart beats faster and blood vessels constrict, which increases peripheral vascular resistance. Under normal circumstances, these cardiac and vascular responses allow a person to maintain normal blood pressure while sitting or standing for an extended time. But for a pregnant woman with hypertension, these mechanisms further elevate blood pressure.

• *Don't lie flat on your back for long periods of time.* In this position, the pregnant woman's uterus lies directly on the vena cava and compresses it. Vena caval compression has several possible consequences. By impairing venous return to the heart, it may trigger vasoconstriction and a blood pressure increase. But vena caval compression can also cause a drop in central blood pressure so severe that the woman becomes nauseated, dizzy, diaphoretic, and air hungry—in other words, she experiences symptoms associated with shock. She can quickly and easily reverse these effects simply by turning onto her left side, which relieves the compression.

In the supine position, a pregnant woman's uterus may also compress the aorta, causing decreased uterine blood flow. When both the vena cava and the aorta are compressed (aortocaval compression) blood flow to and from the uterus and placenta is reduced, possibly jeopardizing the fetus.

The uterus may also compress the renal arteries, causing decreased renal blood flow. Remember, PIH has already reduced renal and uterine blood flow by causing vasoconstriction. Anything that causes further vasoconstriction and reduction in blood flow could worsen your patient's condition.

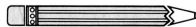

SPECIAL NOTE: Recommend that your patient minimize the length of time she lies on her *right* side. Because the inferior vena cava is located on the right side in some women, a right-side-lying position may also compress the vena cava. But tell her that occasionally resting on her right side is safe, provided she doesn't experience adverse reactions. Teach her the signs and symptoms of vena caval compression, and instruct her to immediately change positions if she experiences them.

• *Do change body positions frequently—as often as possible throughout the day.* If she must stand for prolonged periods, advise her to periodically sit or, if possible, lie down. Skeletal muscle contractions during position changes help reduce venous pooling in her legs and feet.

• *Do lie on your left side when resting.* This is especially important for a woman in her third trimester. By assuming the left lateral position, she displaces the uterus, which relieves pressure on abdominal blood vessels. This, in turn, improves blood flow to the uterus and the kidneys and improves venous return to the heart. Encourage your patient to rest in this position 2 to 3 hours daily.

## CHRONIC HYPERTENSION AND PREGNANCY

If a woman with chronic hypertension becomes pregnant, she's more likely to develop preeclampsia. As you learned on page 102, preeclampsia may jeopardize the fetus by reducing placental blood supply. If preeclampsia develops in addition to preexisting hypertension, the fetus is at special risk of abruptio placentae, along with developmental problems associated with reduced placental blood flow.

If the patient is taking a thiazide diuretic, the doctor will probably continue it. But if she's taking a beta blocker or reserpine, the doctor may discontinue that medication and substitute hydralazine hydrochloride or methyldopa. Why? Because beta blockers may keep the fetus' heart rate from rising if the fetus is stressed; reserpine can cause fetal bradycardia.

Generally, any medication taken during pregnancy is a potential threat to the fetus' health. The best medicine of all, as usual, is prevention. Teach the hypertensive patient to recognize and report signs of preeclampsia.

*Note:* Not all pregnant women with chronic hypertension develop preeclampsia. Remember, blood pressure normally *drops* during pregnancy. In about one third of all pregnant hypertensive patients, blood pressure drops by itself.

# MATERNAL ASSESSMENT

## P.I.H.: RECOGNIZING A PATIENT AT RISK

Early pregnancy-induced hypertension (PIH) is, for the most part, asymptomatic. About the only sign of PIH you'll observe, and the only one your patient is likely to mention, is swelling. During a routine visit, you may notice that her face or hands look somewhat puffy. Or, she may casually mention that her wedding band feels tighter. Unless you recognize these early clues, your patient's PIH can go undetected.

To prevent that possibility, familiarize yourself with the risk factors associated with PIH. Then, carefully review your patient's health history for them.

PIH risk factors include:
• Age extreme (above age 35 or below age 20)
• First pregnancy
• Preexisting hypertension
• History of PIH
• Diabetes mellitus
• Vascular or renal disease
• Hydatidiform mole
• Present pregnancy with twins
• Hydramnios (excessive accumulation of amniotic fluid)
• Obesity
• Below-normal weight
• Poor nutrition
• Several previous pregnancies, especially in combination with other risk factors.

If you determine that your patient is a candidate for PIH, be on the lookout, during each of her routine examinations, for increasing blood pressure measurements, extreme weight gain, and hand or face edema.

Make sure your patient is in the same position each time you check her blood pressure.

If you suspect that she has PIH, test her urine for proteinuria. If the test is positive, alert the doctor at once—proteinuria suggests advanced preeclampsia.

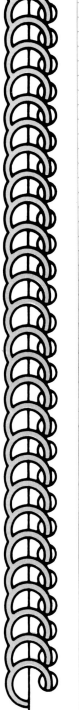

## CRITICAL QUESTIONS

### SPOTTING PREGNANCY-INDUCED HYPERTENSION (P.I.H.)

Ann Draper, age 17, is in her 7th month of pregnancy. She and her husband have been vacationing at a nearby resort for the past week. One afternoon, she arrives in the emergency department with a badly swollen ankle. She tells you she tripped and twisted it while walking.

As you examine her, you note that her blood pressure is elevated, possibly from the pain of her injured ankle. But since she's under 20 and in her last trimester, you know that her high blood pressure could also be an indication of PIH.

Since Ann lives out of town, you can't refer to her medical records for a rundown of her health history. So, in addition to taking a complete Ob history, assess her PIH risk factors by asking her the critical questions listed below.

*Note:* If your patient has PIH, she needs to know how to protect her health during pregnancy. Consider using the handout on the following page as a teaching aid.
• When is your due date? Do you know your most recent blood pressure reading?
• Is this your first pregnancy? If not, how many times have you been pregnant before?
• Are you having any problems with this pregnancy?
• Did you have problems with your other pregnancies? If yes, what were they?
• Have you noticed any swelling in your hands or feet? Or, have your rings felt tighter recently? If yes, when did you first notice these changes?
• How much weight have you gained so far?
• Have you recently been urinating less frequently and in smaller amounts?
• Do you have any medical problems; for example, diabetes or kidney disease?
• Have you ever had high blood pressure?
• Are you currently taking any medication? If so, what kind? What's the dosage? When did you last take a dose?
• Have you ever had seizures or spells?
• Do you smoke?
• Do you have a doctor who has been caring for you during your pregnancy?

## MANAGING PREGNANCY-INDUCED HYPERTENSION AT HOME

You have pregnancy-induced hypertension (PIH), also called preeclampsia. Since your condition is mild, you can manage it at home if you follow the instructions below. Keep in mind, however, that mild PIH can quickly become severe. So follow this home-care plan carefully. Keep regular appointments with your doctor and call him if you have any concerns or questions.

Immediately notify your doctor if you experience severe headaches, dizziness, spots before your eyes, blurred vision, stomach pain, nausea, or vomiting; if you begin urinating only small amounts, or if the baby becomes less active than usual.

Check with your doctor before traveling any distance from home.

Doctor's phone # _____

Nurse's phone # _____

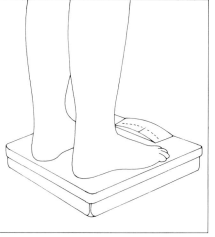

**Activities.** Limit your household activities, such as laundry, housecleaning, and grocery shopping. Sit whenever possible; for example, while you're folding laundry or ironing. Rest in bed at least 1 hour daily. Be sure to lie on your left side while resting.

**Diet.** Eat high protein foods (about 70 to 80 g daily) in addition to regular servings of bread and vegetables. High protein foods include meat, fish, poultry, eggs, milk, cheese, and nuts. (Don't limit your salt intake unless your doctor advises you to.)

Weigh yourself every day before breakfast and record your weight. Notify the doctor or me if you gain 3 to 4 lb (1.36 to 1.81 kg) in 1 week.

**Urine testing.** Test your urine for protein twice a day (a.m. and p.m.), using the test strips I've given you. Be sure to perform the test in a well-lighted room so you can clearly see the color changes on the strip.

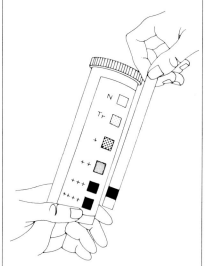

Before starting the test, wash your hands thoroughly with soap and water. Then wash your genital area with soap and water; rinse it and dry it completely with a towel.

Collect a midstream urine specimen in a clean container, and dip the test strip into the specimen. Compare the color changes on the strip with the table of values on your test strip bottle. Notify your doctor or me immediately if your test results are 3+ or 4+.

*Important:* Avoid drinking a lot of water before the test. Water dilutes your urine and may produce false-low results.

# FETAL ASSESSMENT

## ASSESSING THE FETUS

To determine how PIH is affecting the fetus, the doctor will rely on results from one or more of the following assessment tests.

**Ultrasound (ultrasonography).** This test helps determine fetal age, physical development, the amount of amniotic fluid, and placental placement. The test is important for women with PIH, since hypertension can interfere with the normal functions of the placenta. By measuring fetal structures with high frequency sound waves, ultrasound can detect fetal growth retardation and decreased amniotic fluid, which may result from PIH.

**Nonstress test.** This test, which may be done weekly after 32 weeks of gestation, uses ultrasound and phonocardiography to evaluate fetal heart rate (FHR) acceleration in response to fetal movement. Normally, fetal movement triggers the sympathetic nervous system, which increases (accelerates) fetal heart rate. This is a normal (reactive) finding, indicating a nondepressed fetal central nervous system (CNS).

Although standards vary among institutions, generally accepted criteria for normal results are an increase in FHR of 10 beats/minute for at least 15 seconds following fetal movement. Abnormal (nonreactive) findings show little or no increase in FHR following fetal movement and may indicate a CNS problem, hypoxia, acidosis, the influence of narcotics or sedatives, or a sleeping fetus. To confirm abnormal findings, repeat the nonstress test the next day.

**Contraction stress test (oxytocin challenge test).** The doctor will order this test if nonstress test results are nonreactive. Uterine contractions are produced by intravenous administration of oxytocin or by nipple stimulation.

### Fetal heart rate (FHR) variability

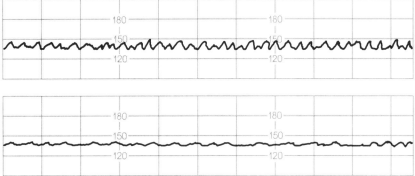

The first graph above shows normal FHR variability, an indicator of fetal well-being, during a contraction stress test. Decreased variability (see the second graph) is indicated by flattening of the waveform. This suggests hypoxia or CNS depression.

Electronic monitoring equipment measures FHR and uterine activity. Results help the doctor evaluate placental function based on the presence or absence of late FHR decelerations (decreased FHR) during a contraction.

Normal findings show no change in FHR or deceleration only at the onset of a contraction, indicating that the fetus will probably do well for another week. Abnormal findings show either late decelerations (a decrease in FHR after the peak of the contraction) or variable decelerations, indicating impaired placental function. Placental impairment may deprive the fetus of oxygen, leading to fetal acidosis and asphyxia.

Closely monitor the patient during and after the test for premature labor. *Note:* Contraction stress tests have a high false-positive rate. Consider other assessment findings before drawing conclusions.

**Estriol/creatinine excretion (E/C ratio).** This 24-hour urine test determines the ratio between estriol and creatinine in urine. This test reflects the placenta's ability to convert dehydroisoandrosterone (a substance secreted by the fetus' adrenal glands) into estriol, which is then excreted in the mother's urine.

Estriol levels normally increase as pregnancy progresses; creatinine levels remain constant. In a normal pregnancy, estriol levels increase from about 12 mg/24 hours to about 30 mg/24 hours at term. Estriol values of less than 4 mg/24 hours at any point in the pregnancy—or those which show a drop of 50% or more from the previous reading—may indicate severe fetal compromise or death. A drop of 35% from the average of three previous consecutive readings is also cause for concern and further testing.

**Amniocentesis.** This test assesses fetal lung maturity and the presence of meconium staining the amniotic fluid. Fetal lung development is indicated by the presence of two pulmonary surface-active substances—lecithin and sphingomyelin. Their relative proportions, called the L/S ratio, are normally 2:1 after 37 weeks of gestation. An L/S ratio greater than 2:1 before 33 weeks can indicate accelerated lung maturity, a possible effect of PIH. This ratio indicates that a newborn infant delivered before term is unlikely to develop respiratory distress syndrome. Meconium staining at any time can indicate fetal distress and the need for further study or immediate delivery.

# P.I.H. MANAGEMENT

## CARING FOR THE PATIENT WITH SEVERE PREECLAMPSIA

Jane Mercer, age 32, is due to deliver her first child in a month. Three weeks ago, Jane was diagnosed as having mild preeclampsia. Since then, she's effectively managed her condition at home—until today, that is. Jane awoke this morning with a headache and her blood pressure was elevated (142/92 mm Hg). As the day progressed, she began feeling dizzy and nauseated. When she took her blood pressure again that evening, it was even higher (148/96 mm Hg). Realizing that Jane's condition was worsening, her husband drove her to the hospital, where she was admitted for treatment of severe preeclampsia.

Now Jane's arrived on your unit and you're responsible for planning her care. Remember, your major objective is to prevent severe preeclampsia from progressing to eclampsia (seizures), which can kill both mother and fetus. To do that, your care plan should include these steps:
• Put the patient in a quiet room—preferably a single room. Because she's hyperirritable and her central nervous system is unstable, any sudden noise or movement—even flicking a light off or on—could trigger a convulsion.
• Confine the patient to bed rest. Encourage her to lie in the left lateral position as much as possible, to prevent vena caval compression by the uterus (see page 104). Keep her under close observation.
• In case of seizure or cardiac arrest, keep emergency equipment and drugs on hand. You need resuscitative equipment, an oral airway, suction equipment, and special emergency drugs (diazepam, calcium gluconate, and magnesium sulfate).
• Administer medications, as or-

dered. *Important:* Always assess the patient's vital signs before giving any medication.
• Frequently check her vision, level of consciousness, and deep tendon reflexes. Immediately notify the doctor of any changes. If she's receiving magnesium sulfate, absent patellar reflexes indicate magnesium toxicity.
• Pad her side rails to protect her from injury if she has a seizure.
• Every 4 hours (or more frequently), monitor her blood pressure, pulse rate, respiratory rate, fetal heart tones, urine output, and urine protein level. Immediately report any changes to the doctor.
• Assess the patient's fluid balance by measuring her intake and output and by weighing her daily.
• Stay alert for fetal distress by closely monitoring the results of stress and nonstress tests, and the patient's serial serum or urinary estriol levels.

Because your patient requires careful monitoring, you'll be performing numerous nursing procedures throughout the day. Since these procedures can interfere with her rest and increase her anxiety, try to limit the interruptions by performing several procedures together at various times of the day.

But don't limit your contact with her so much that she feels isolated or neglected. Remember, she's probably very anxious. Spend a few minutes after you've completed your nursing care to talk with her and answer her questions. Keep her informed about the fetus' condition. She needs your continuing emotional support.

## DRUG THERAPY: WEIGHING FETAL RISK

Before the doctor prescribes a drug to treat PIH, he'll weigh the potential benefits to the patient against possible risks for the fetus both before and immediately after birth. The following chart details possible fetal adverse reactions associated with several commonly prescribed drugs.

### ANTICONVULSANTS

**diazepam**
*Adverse effect:* Hemorrhage (in the fetus)

**magnesium sulfate**
*Adverse effects:* Sedation or respiratory depression, magnesium toxicity (in the neonate)

### ANTIHYPERTENSIVES

**hydralazine hydrochloride**
*Adverse effect:* Tachycardia (in the fetus)

**methyldopa**
*Adverse effects:* Hemolytic anemia (in the fetus), meconium ileus (in the neonate)

**reserpine**
*Adverse effects:* Upper airway stuffiness, respiratory depression, lethargy, anorexia, galactorrhea, bradycardia (in the fetus)

### THIAZIDE DIURETICS

**hydrochlorothiazide**
*Adverse effects:* Thrombocytopenia, hypokalemia, jaundice, hyponatremia (in the fetus)

# P.I.H. MANAGEMENT

## ADMINISTERING MAGNESIUM SULFATE

To protect the fetus, the doctor will try to avoid treating PIH with drugs. But if a pregnant patient has severe preeclampsia and conservative measures haven't helped, he may prescribe magnesium sulfate (MgSO$_4$), an anticonvulsant, to prevent seizures. (As an alternative, he may attempt to lower blood pressure by ordering an antihypertensive drug such as hydralazine hydrochloride, a sedative, or a thiazide diuretic.)

### MAGNESIUM SULFATE (MgSO$_4$)

A cerebral depressant. Replaces calcium at the myoneural junction, reducing neuromuscular irritability, relaxing vascular smooth muscle, and causing vasodilation.

**Dosage**

*I.M.:* 5 to 10 g of 25% to 50% solution every 4 hours for a maximum of 6 doses. Because of the large dosage involved, divide each dose and give half in each buttock. *I.V. bolus:* 1 to 4 g of 10% to 25% solution, at a rate no faster than 1.5 ml/minute for a 10% solution. *I.V. infusion:* loading dose of 4 g of 50% solution in 250 ml dextrose 5% in water over 15 minutes; then maintenance dose of 1 to 2 g/hour. *Maximum rate:* 3 ml/minute.

**Contraindications**

Use with *extreme caution* if the patient has impaired renal function, myocardial damage, or heart block; or if she's in labor.

**Onset and duration**

*I.M.:* 1 hour onset, lasts 3 to 4 hours. *I.V.:* immediate onset, lasts about 30 minutes.

**Possible adverse reactions**

Sweating, flushing, burning sensation (with rapid I.V. infusion), drowsiness, transient paralysis, depressed reflexes, hypothermia, hypotension, circulatory collapse, heart block, nausea, respiratory paralysis, hypocalcemia

**Special considerations**

• Check hospital policy for guidelines before giving MgSO$_4$.
• Use cautiously with digoxin; monitor for dysrhythmias.
• If the patient's taking barbiturates, narcotics, hypnotics, or systemic anesthetic agents, be aware of additive depressant effects.
• Avoid administering MgSO$_4$ within 2 hours before delivery. Magnesium toxicity may cause hypotonia or respiratory distress in the newborn.
• Test the patellar reflex before administering each dose (or hourly during a continuous infusion). If the reflex is absent, hold the dose and notify the doctor. An absent patellar reflex may indicate toxicity.
• Monitor vital signs every 15 to 30 minutes during continuous I.V. infusion, and before each dose if giving intermittently.
• Monitor intake and output. If urine output is less than 30 ml/hour, contact the doctor.
• Hold the drug and notify the doctor if the patient's respiratory rate falls below 14 breaths/minute.
• Warn the patient that she may feel nauseated temporarily.
• Change the needle after drawing the solution into the syringe for I.M. injection. If ordered, add 1 to 2 ml of 1% procaine hydrochloride or lidocaine hydrochloride to reduce pain at the injection site.
• For I.M. injection give deep I.M., using the Z-track technique. Rotate the needle like a wheel during the injection.
• Check serum magnesium levels as ordered. Therapeutic range is 2.5 to 7.5 mg/dl. Patient should not receive more than 40 g daily.
• Keep a syringe and an ampule of calcium gluconate on hand, to reverse magnesium toxicity if necessary. Administer 10 to 20 ml of 10% solution I.V. over 20 minutes (0.5 ml/minute).

## ECLAMPSIA: EMERGENCY CARE

Consider this situation: Your patient, 36-year-old Sharon Mitchell, is hospitalized for severe preeclampsia. That afternoon, she has a seizure. Because Mrs. Mitchell has no history of seizures, you know she's become eclamptic. Act quickly, following the steps below.

**During the seizure**

• Don't leave the patient. Call for help and have someone notify the doctor.
• Try to maintain a patent airway and reduce the risk of aspiration by turning her head to one side. But never *force* her head in any direction. Use a suction catheter through her nose to clear her oropharynx of secretions. *Caution:* Don't force any object, including a tongue depressor, between the patient's clenched teeth.
• Administer oxygen.
• Protect her from harming herself. Pad the side rails, if they aren't already padded.
• Establish an I.V. line (if necessary) and administer magnesium sulfate. For persistent seizures, give amobarbital sodium or diazepam, as ordered.

**Follow-up care**

• Check the patient's vital signs and neurologic responses every 15 minutes.
• Monitor the fetal heartbeat with an electronic monitor or stethoscope.
• Insert an indwelling (Foley) catheter, if necessary, to monitor fluid output. Document intake and output meticulously.
• Reduce disturbances. Place the patient in a quiet, dark room or shade her eyes and cover her ears. Bright lights, loud noises, and sudden movements may induce another seizure.
• Record details about the seizure and any subsequent ones. Include information about the duration and characteristics of the

convulsion and fetal status. If a coma followed, include information about its depth and duration.
• Watch for signs and symptoms of cerebral hemorrhage, abruptio placentae (such as vaginal bleeding, uterine tenderness, change in fetal activity or heart rate, or sustained abdominal pain), pulmonary edema, and cardiac failure.
• Assess for uterine contractions and signs of labor.
• Be prepared to send the patient to the delivery room for induction of labor or for a cesarean section. (Expect to wait 4 to 6 hours for the patient and fetus to stabilize.)
• Be prepared to transfer the patient to the intensive care unit or to a tertiary care hospital.

## Emotional support

Keep in mind that the patient has had a harrowing experience. Although you may become preoccupied with providing nursing care, don't overlook her psychological needs. Give plenty of support and reassurance to the patient and her family.

Following the seizure, the patient may experience a period of amnesia. Explain to her and her family what happened. Inform them about the fetus' status as well, and answer their questions.

The patient may be transferred to a high-risk center. If so, she'll probably be frightened and confused, and may possibly feel guilty about endangering her baby. Take steps to reduce her anxiety and make the transfer as smooth as possible.

## AFTER DELIVERY: YOUR ROLE

After giving birth, your PIH patient remains at risk of developing seizures and other complications. Closely monitor her condition for the first 48 hours, keeping the following points in mind.

**Postpartum care.** The patient's doctor will probably continue antihypertensive medication until her diastolic blood pressure falls below 110 mm Hg. He may also keep her on magnesium sulfate for 24 hours after her blood pressure drops, to reduce the risk of a seizure.

Monitor her condition by documenting her vital signs, deep tendon reflexes (especially the patellar reflex), and fluid intake and output every 4 hours. Her blood pressure may remain high for a few days following delivery but will probably revert to normal within 10 to 14 days. Or, her blood pressure may remain at mildly preeclamptic levels for 6 to 8 weeks after delivery.

Stay alert for a sudden blood pressure drop accompanied by decreased urinary output and in-

"Once eclampsia develops, the prognosis for both mother and fetus is poor. That's why the nurse's role in identifying and managing preeclampsia is absolutely crucial.

"Emotional support for the preeclamptic patient is important, too. She's likely to feel guilty and anxious when she realizes that her body has become a hostile environment for her baby."

**Betty Glenn Harris, RN, PhD**
Assistant Professor, Undergraduate Obstetrics, University of North Carolina School of Nursing, Chapel Hill

creased pulse rate. This combination may indicate hemorrhage and impending shock.

*An eclamptic patient loses almost twice as much blood as the normal pregnant patient during the postpartum period. As a result, she's at greater risk of cardiovascular or renal complications— especially since she's already hypovolemic from having PIH.*

Finally, watch for postpartum diuresis, which could lower serum magnesium levels and cause seizures.

**The long-term prognosis.** Expect your patient to be concerned about how PIH will affect her health and subsequent pregnancies, if she plans to have more children. Tell her that although hypertension-related problems aren't inevitable, her risk of developing chronic hypertension or PIH during future pregnancies is higher than average. Stress the importance of regular blood pressure monitoring to check for hypertension, and prenatal care if she becomes pregnant again.

If your patient had eclampsia, inform her that these factors increase her odds of developing PIH in later pregnancies:
• obesity
• hypertension persisting through the 10th day after delivery
• onset of preeclampsia before the 36th week of gestation
• an average systolic blood pressure of over 160 mm Hg during eclampsia.

Urge her to continue regular medical care if any of these factors is present.

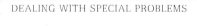

# PHEOCHROMOCYTOMA

## ANOTHER KIND OF HYPERTENSION

"Lately, it seems as if I'm unusually jumpy. Even my wife's commented on it," says Ted Freeman. "And I've been having a lot of headaches, too."

A 38-year-old high school physics teacher and basketball coach, Mr. Freeman has been admitted to your hospital for testing. While taking his health history, you learn that his blood pressure measured 160/100 during a recent physical. Although the examination revealed no other trouble signs, Mr. Freeman is uneasy. "I've had three or four spells where I felt really funny," he tells you. "All of them happened during close games, when I was pretty excited. My head was pounding, I could feel my heart racing, and I couldn't catch my breath. When I told the doctor about these spells, he said he'd better do some tests."

As you're weighing him, Mr. Freeman mentions that he's lost weight recently. When you take his pulse, you notice his palms are damp. Mr. Freeman's history and symptoms make you suspect pheochromocytoma—and the 24-hour urine specimen request noted on his admission order tells you that the doctor suspects the same thing.

Urine that's high in catecholamines suggests the existence of a pheochromocytoma: a type of tumor that releases excessive epinephrine and norepinephrine, causing chronic vasoconstriction. Most pheochromocytomas grow in the adrenal medulla. If this proves to be the case with Mr. Freeman, the doctor will probably perform an adrenalectomy to remove the tumor. After surgery, chances are good that your patient's hypertension will vanish.

Read on to learn more about the adrenal glands.

## A LOOK AT THE ADRENAL GLANDS

Two small, yellowish, pyramidal structures—the adrenal glands—cap the kidneys. Each gland consists of an outer layer, the adrenal cortex, enclosing an inner layer, the adrenal medulla. The cortex synthesizes three types of steroid hormones (glucocorticoids, mineralocorticoids, and androgens) and the medulla produces two catecholamines (epinephrine and norepinephrine). For details, read what follows.

**Adrenal cortex.** In response to the adrenocorticotropic hormone (ACTH) secreted by the pituitary gland, the adrenal cortex releases three groups of hormones. The *glucocorticoids* (primarily cortisol) are vital to metabolism. They aid in the breakdown of protein into amino acids, helping to produce glucose (thereby influencing blood sugar levels). Among other functions, they reduce the inflammatory response to infection.

Aldosterone, the most important of the *mineralocorticoids,* promotes reabsorption of sodium and excretion of potassium. Because this process increases plasma volume, excessive aldosterone secretion can cause hypertension.

The *androgens* control the development of secondary sex characteristics.

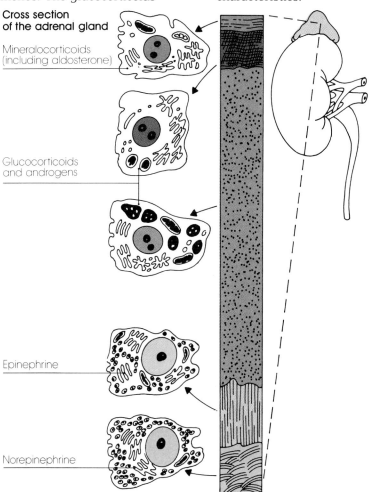

**Cross section of the adrenal gland**

Mineralocorticoids (including aldosterone)

Glucocorticoids and androgens

Epinephrine

Norepinephrine

**Adrenal medulla.** The adrenal medulla, site of most (but not all) pheochromocytomas, responds directly to impulses from the sympathetic nervous system (SNS) and from the hypothalamus. It produces two catecholamine hormones. *Epinephrine* (also called adrenaline) acts to:
• increase the heart's rate and force of contraction
• raise blood sugar levels by stimulating the liver to turn glycogen into glucose
• constrict kidney vessels, which slows urine production.

*Norepinephrine* (also called noradrenaline) is produced by SNS cells elsewhere in the body, as well as by the adrenal medulla. Among other functions, it acts to:
• constrict arteries, raising arterial blood pressure
• constrict veins, improving venous return to the heart
• constrict peripheral vessels, increasing peripheral resistance and raising systolic blood pressure. In an emergency, peripheral vasoconstriction channels blood away from the skin, extremities, and bowel and toward the vital organs.

**A delicate balance.** Looking at each hormone's job, you can see that an overproduction of any one throws the body's functions out of balance. Too much aldosterone causes the body to retain sodium, leading to fluid retention and hypertension. Too much glucocorticoid secretion increases blood sugar to diabetic levels, as does too much epinephrine. Epinephrine can also overstimulate the heart, leading to dysrhythmias, and increase the metabolic rate to a point where the cells exhaust their oxygen supply and switch to anaerobic metabolism. Too much of the vasoconstrictor norepinephrine raises blood pressure beyond safe levels.

## SIGNS AND SYMPTOMS: REASONS FOR SUSPICION

Except for elevated blood pressure, the physical examination of a patient with pheochromocytoma is likely to be unremarkable. That's why a thorough health history—with special attention to symptoms your patient experiences—may be the key to identifying this condition.

If your hypertensive patient reports recurring symptoms, such as severe headaches, profuse sweating, and nausea, take special note. These are a few cardinal symptoms of *paroxysms of hypertension*. Although not all patients with pheochromocytoma experience paroxysms, they're considered a classic sign of the disease.

**Signs of paroxysm.** During a paroxysm, the patient typically suffers an intense headache, profuse sweating, palpitations, and anxiety or nervousness, often with chest or abdominal pain, nausea, vomiting, and flushed or pale skin. Blood pressure and heart rate often rise to alarming levels, and vision may blur. A paroxysm, which may last a few minutes, a few hours, or longer, occasionally leads to stroke.

Usually, paroxysms occur at intervals of days or weeks. For some patients, however, they occur as frequently as 25 times a day. A precipitating factor may be identifiable: position change, pressure on the tumor, emotional upset, or reaction to certain medications, such as epinephrine or histamine. Often, however, the crisis is apparently spontaneous, with no recognizable cause. In time, these crises become more frequent, more severe, and more lengthy.

**Other signs.** Even if your patient doesn't experience paroxysms, he may report one or more of the associated symptoms. Or, he may report one or more of the following:
• dyspnea
• postural hypotension
• angina
• weight loss
• epigastric pain
• constipation
• carbohydrate intolerance
• fever
• cold, clammy skin
• paresthesias.

## DIAGNOSTIC TESTS: WHAT TO EXPECT

If the doctor suspects pheochromocytoma, he'll take several steps, as detailed below.

**Confirming the diagnosis.** First, the doctor orders assays of the patient's urine—a 24-hour specimen, if possible. If the tumor is present, the urine will contain elevated levels of vanillylmandelic acid (VMA), catecholamines, and metanephrines (see page 39 for normal values).

Pharmacologic diagnostic tests—administration of a provocative agent, such as histamine, tyramine, or glucagon; or of the alpha blocker phentol-amine—are rare today. Test results are significantly less reliable than urine assay results—and the test itself may alter blood pressure dangerously.

**Determining location.** Once the doctor's determined that a tumor's present, he needs to pinpoint its location. Although 90% of all pheochromocytomas occur in the adrenal medulla, the doctor will order further testing to make certain that his patient isn't among the 10% with extra-adrenal tumors. (Urine test results may give a hint. Strong

CONTINUED ON PAGE 114

# PHEOCHROMOCYTOMA

## DIAGNOSTIC TESTS: WHAT TO EXPECT CONTINUED

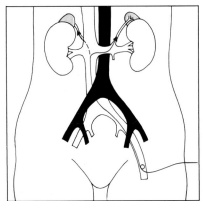

**Renal vein sampling**
During this diagnostic test, a catheter is inserted into one of the femoral veins, advanced through the vena cava, and threaded into each adrenal vein. Blood specimens are obtained and tested for catecholamine content.

predominance of norepinephrine over epinephrine suggests an extraadrenal tumor.)

Chances are, the doctor will order a *computerized tomography (CT) scan*. This noninvasive procedure has a 91% success rate in locating even small tumors.

If your hospital doesn't have a CT scanner, the doctor has several other options. Each alternative, however, has disadvantages.

*Ultrasound* can pick up only tumors that are at least 2 cm in diameter—larger than many pheochromocytomas.

*Angiography*—radiographic visualization—is an accurate but risky invasive procedure, since the contrast medium sometimes precipitates hypertensive crisis.

*Selective catheterizing and sampling* of adrenal veins, the inferior vena cava, and abdominal veins for catecholamine content is another way to locate very small or multiple tumors. Because this test is less risky than angiography, the doctor may order it to check for tumors that a CT scan has failed to locate.

## UNDERSTANDING SURGICAL RISKS

When deciding to perform surgery, the doctor will take precautions to minimize the patient's risk. Here are a few points he'll consider.

**Blood pressure: The first concern.** Hypertensive crisis and hypotensive shock are both dangers during an adrenalectomy. The doctor may delay surgery until drug therapy has stabilized the patient's blood pressure at or near normal levels; even so, continuous blood pressure and heart rate monitoring during surgery is crucial, and the doctor may order intraoperative drug management as well. Induction of anesthesia, intubation, and manipulation of the tumor may send the patient's blood pressure shooting up, while loss of fluid and removal of the tumor that had been causing the initial hypertension may make his blood pressure plummet.

**Hemorrhage: Another hazard.** Since the adrenal glands are highly vascular, hemorrhage is another major risk during adrenalectomy. The surgeon may order preoperative administration of 1 or 2 units of blood, to counter expected blood loss.

A multitude of small vessels surround each adrenal gland; all need ligation to prevent excessive bleeding. Securing the right adrenal vein is particularly important, since it's directly connected to the vena cava.

The common hepatic duct and the spleen are so close to the right and the left adrenal glands (respectively) that they may be damaged during resection. Any of these injuries could cause postoperative hemorrhage and shock.

**The odds for success.** If the pheochromocytoma is benign, complete removal cures hypertension in about 75% of all patients. Recurring hypertension in

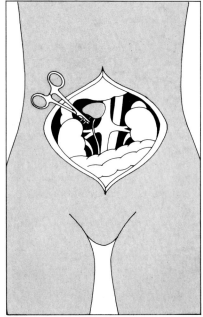

**Anterior abdominal approach**
Eight or nine times out of ten, pheochromocytoma develops within the medulla of one adrenal gland (usually the right). But bilateral adrenal lesions and extraadrenal lesions—some of them multiple—do occur, even in cases where a CT scan has identified only one tumor. So the surgeon will probably use an anterior abdominal approach that allows him to look for additional lesions in the surrounding area.

the other 25% usually responds well to standard drug management.

If the tumor is malignant—about 10% are— it will metastasize to the lymph nodes, liver, lungs, or bone in 5 to 10 years after the original tumor is removed. No radiation or chemotherapy treatments have proven effective in controlling such metastasis. However, since death usually results from hypertension, rather than from the malignancy, drug therapy may provide the patient with several more productive years of life. The drug regimen usually includes alpha and beta blockers for direct blood pressure control and metyrosine to inhibit catecholamine synthesis by the metastasized tumor.

## TEACHING YOUR PATIENT ABOUT SURGERY

If your patient is facing surgery, he's understandably worried—maybe so worried that he'll have a hard time absorbing much of what you tell him.

To reduce his anxiety, answer his questions first. Then, let him know what will be happening to him before, during, and after surgery, and encourage him to ask more questions. (Be alert for nonverbal reactions, too.) Do your best to communicate your concern for how he's feeling and thinking.

Include your patient's family in your teaching sessions, if possible. They're worried, too—and they're potential allies in your effort to help your patient help himself. Let them know that their support is important to the recovery process—not only their emotional support, but also their assistance in persuading the patient to perform coughing, deep breathing, and leg exercises during the postoperative period.

Take care to inform your patient about where he'll be going following surgery and what will be happening to him. For example, if he'll go to the ICU after surgery, explain what to expect. If possible, arrange for a tour of the ICU or a visit from an ICU nurse.

Use the following as a reminder of some important points to cover.

### The day before surgery
• The surgical prep procedure (including shaving his chest or abdomen, if necessary)
• The sedative he'll receive before going to bed
• Why eating and drinking aren't allowed after midnight
• The coughing, deep breathing, and leg exercises you'll ask him to do postoperatively
• Family visiting before and after surgery (as hospital rules permit).

### The morning of surgery
• The need to remove dentures, prostheses, and jewelry (except a plain wedding band, if he wears one, that you'll tape securely to his finger)
• Preanesthetic procedures and medication. Tell him that you'll ask him to urinate and put on a clean hospital gown before giving him a preoperative sedative.
• Holding-area procedures, including I.V. fluid administration

---

*Many hospitals have films or pamphlets that can help you prepare the patient for his surgical experience. Make use of these materials if they're available.*

---

• Entering the operating room. Explain that he'll be transferred from the stretcher to the operating table and securely strapped in place. Because of preanesthetic medications, however, he may be unaware of these events.
• Waking up in the recovery room—with I.V., nasogastric tube, and indwelling (Foley) catheter in place. Since he may still be intubated when he wakes up, prepare him for this. Explain that the recovery room nurses will closely monitor his condition and take his vital signs every 5 to 15 minutes.
• His return to his room.

*Note:* Your patient may experience postoperative pain. Assure him that he'll have medication to ease it.

## BEFORE SURGERY: NURSING CONSIDERATIONS

Teaching isn't your only preoperative responsibility. In addition, you must alter the patient's treatment regimen, as ordered, to prepare him for surgery. For instance, the doctor may change the patient's drug order or prescribe an increase in salt intake, to increase blood volume.

Monitor your patient closely for alterations in his condition. Keep an eye on his weight and blood sugar levels as well as his blood pressure, since diabetes mellitus is a possible complication of pheochromocytoma.

The day before surgery, be sure staff members on the night shift know that the patient can take nothing by mouth after midnight. Also, remind the patient about this, and take away his water pitcher.

On the day of surgery, complete your patient teaching by answering any last-minute questions your patient has. If he has a remaining doubt or misunderstanding that you can't clear up to his satisfaction or if he gives you any reason to suspect that his consent isn't well-informed, notify the doctor and document your findings.

Then, complete all preoperative procedures, using your hospital's preoperative checklist as a guide. Initial each step on the list as you complete the procedure.

*Important:* Document test results *before* checking them off. If another staff member performs a step, ask her to initial it.

Include the checklist in the paperwork that you send to the OR with the patient, to give the OR nurse a convenient means to double-check that all procedures were completed.

## DEEP BREATHING AND COUGHING

After surgery, deep breathing and coughing are important parts of the recovery process. By doing these two exercises every 2 hours after surgery, you'll expand your lungs and keep them free of fluid. The following procedure will help you do the right kind of deep breathing and coughing—using your diaphragm and abdominal muscles.

Practice these exercises two or three times a day before surgery, so that you'll find them easier to do after surgery. Use this aid to remind yourself what to do.

**1** Lie comfortably on your back, with your knees slightly flexed. Raise the head of your bed (or ask the nurse to raise it for you). Put a pillow over your abdomen and lace your fingers together on top of the pillow, as shown here. This is called *splinting*. By supporting your incision this way, you'll reduce the discomfort you may feel right after surgery.

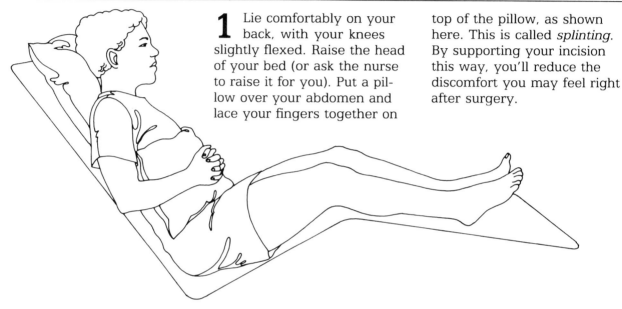

**2** Breathe out normally. Now, close your mouth and breathe in deeply through your nose. While you're doing this, concentrate on what your hands are doing. If you feel them rising, you're breathing correctly.

When you've taken in all the air you can, hold your breath and slowly count to five.

**3** Purse your lips as you would to whistle and let all the air out through your mouth, without puffing your cheeks. Use your abdominal muscles to squeeze out every last bit of air that you can. You'll feel your ribs sink downward and inward.

**4** Now, take another deep breath. This time, hold it. Then, cough—a good, sharp cough. Concentrate on feeling your diaphragm force all the air out of your chest.

Do these exercises at least two more times.

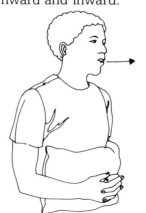

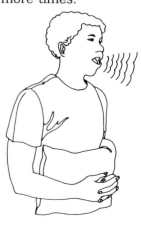

# POSTOP CARE

## GIVING POSTOPERATIVE CARE

Your patient's blood pressure may rise or fall sharply after surgery. For the first 24 hours, he'll probably remain in the recovery room or the intensive care unit, where his blood pressure and urine output can be monitored constantly. Here's a summary of the care he'll need.

**The first few hours.** As soon as your patient responds when spoken to, start him on the coughing and deep-breathing exercises you taught him. Every couple of hours, ask him to flex each foot 5 to 10 times by pointing the toe up toward his knee and then down toward the foot of the bed. Also ask him to flex and then straighten his legs.

Monitor your patient's pain level carefully. As ordered, give him analgesics while the pain is still relatively mild. Don't wait for it to peak.

The doctor may order corticosteroids—intravenously or intramuscularly at first, orally later—to replace those the removed adrenal gland no longer supplies. Monitor your patient for the subtle signs of corticosteroid imbalance that can precede shock: dehydration, restlessness, tachycardia. (Keep in mind, however, that these signs and symptoms can also reflect pain and other problems.)

Since corticosteroids suppress such usual signs of infection as inflammation, watch the incision site carefully. Use strict aseptic technique during every dressing change.

**Continuing recovery.** Your patient will probably stay on bed rest until his blood pressure stabilizes. Begin ambulating him as soon as the doctor permits, and encourage the patient to resume his normal activities as soon as he can comfortably do so.

If his corticosteroid therapy is continuing, make sure he understands that the drug is correcting a temporary shortage (unless, of course, he had a bilateral adrenalectomy). When his body is again maintaining adequate hormone levels, the doctor will discontinue the drug.

Though your patient probably won't have further problems, tell him to let his doctor know if any characteristic symptoms (see page 113) return when he's under stress. And encourage him to wear a medic-alert tag identifying the therapy he's undergone.

### Postoperative foot and leg exercises

By flexing his knee and lifting his leg, the postoperative patient helps promote circulation and maintain muscle tone in his leg.

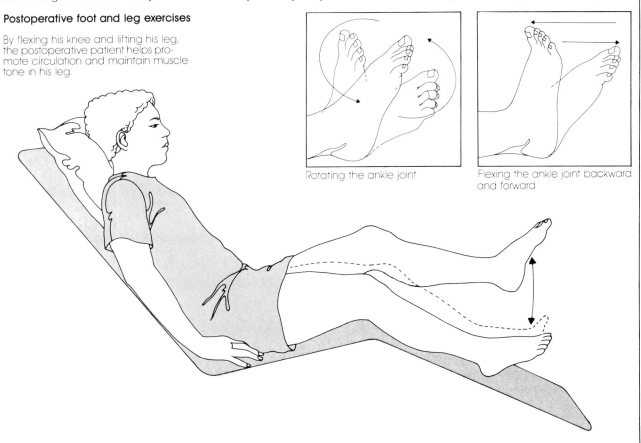

Rotating the ankle joint

Flexing the ankle joint backward and forward

# HEMORRHAGIC STROKE

## UNDERSTANDING HEMORRHAGIC STROKE

Hemorrhagic stroke, one of the most devastating consequences of uncontrolled hypertension, is caused by a break in one of the brain's blood vessels (usually an artery) deep within brain tissue. Bleeding is often massive and may follow a sudden blood pressure increase triggered by sneezing, coughing, or straining. Blood seeps out of the damaged artery, causing displacement and compression of adjacent tissues. The result: ischemia or death of brain cells.

Depending on the size of the bleed and the amount of compression, intracranial pressure may rise dangerously. This leads first to a shift of structures from the midline, and eventually to brain herniation and massive brain cell destruction.

Although the exact cause of vessel rupture is unknown, several possibilities exist. For example, hemorrhage may result when an arterial wall becomes weakened by arteriosclerosis secondary to hypertension. Under these circumstances, any sudden increase in blood pressure could cause a rupture.

According to another theory, the initial event is a spasm of the cerebral artery, causing ischemia and tissue softening in the area of the spasm. If the spasm continues, necrosis of the blood vessel wall occurs, leading to vessel wall breakdown and bleeding.

Yet another possible cause of bleeding is rupture resulting from small malformations of the cerebral vessels.

Whatever the underlying cause, hemorrhagic stroke has a high mortality rate. Read the following pages to learn more about this life-threatening complication.

## SITES AND SIGNS OF HEMORRHAGIC STROKE

Hemorrhagic stroke from hypertension generally originates in one of five areas of the brain. Because each area of the brain controls different neurologic functions, your assessment findings will vary accordingly.

For a close look at these variations, refer to the illustration below. As you see, it lists the five most common bleeding sites and the signs and symptoms characteristic of bleeding at each site. Study it carefully.

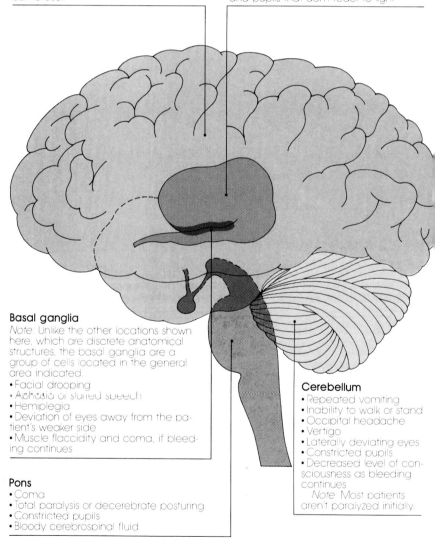

### Cerebral cortex
• Seizures
• Hemiparesis (more severe in arm than leg, if hemorrhage is in frontal lobe)
  *Note*: Most patients don't become comatose.

### Thalamus
• Hemiplegia or hemiparesis
• Aphasia possible
• Ocular disturbances, including downward deviating eyes, unequal pupils, and pupils that don't react to light

### Basal ganglia
*Note*: Unlike the other locations shown here, which are discrete anatomical structures, the basal ganglia are a group of cells located in the general area indicated.
• Facial drooping
• Aphasia or slurred speech
• Hemiplegia
• Deviation of eyes away from the patient's weaker side
• Muscle flaccidity and coma, if bleeding continues

### Pons
• Coma
• Total paralysis or decerebrate posturing
• Constricted pupils
• Bloody cerebrospinal fluid

### Cerebellum
• Repeated vomiting
• Inability to walk or stand
• Occipital headache
• Vertigo
• Laterally deviating eyes
• Constricted pupils
• Decreased level of consciousness as bleeding continues
  *Note*: Most patients aren't paralyzed initially.

## HEMORRHAGIC STROKE: A CASE IN POINT

Louis Scanlon, age 54, is the senior accountant for a fast-growing computer company. He's just been carried into the emergency department by two of his co-workers who tell you that he's unable to stand or walk and has been vomiting repeatedly for about an hour. Though his speech is slurred, Mr. Scanlon manages to explain that he felt dizzy when he arrived at work that morning, then developed a headache at the back of his head that worsened as the morning progressed. By lunchtime, he was too weak and dizzy to stand. Until this morning he'd been feeling fine, except for some fatigue from working extra hours to complete the company's annual audit.

Upon questioning Mr. Scanlon about his health history, you learn that he's had hypertension for about 3 years and has been taking medication for it. When you ask him if he takes his medication regularly, however, he concedes that he's taken it sporadically for the past year, because he's felt fine.

Significant assessment findings include elevated blood pressure (178/106 mm Hg), laterally deviating eyes, and constricted pupils. These findings, along with his health history and your observations, lead you to suspect that Mr. Scanlon is a victim of a cerebellar hemorrhagic stroke.

## PINPOINTING THE PROBLEM

To arrive at a final diagnosis for a suspected stroke patient, the doctor needs to identify the exact site and extent of any bleeding that may have occurred in the patient's brain. The quickest and most accurate way to obtain this information is with a computerized tomography (CT) scan (see illustration at right). If your hospital doesn't have a CT scanner, the doctor will rely on a lumbar puncture, skull X-rays, blood work, and possibly an arteriogram to evaluate the patient's intracranial status.

If a hemorrhage has occurred, cerebrospinal fluid (CSF) may be bloody and CSF pressure may be high. If the hemorrhage is

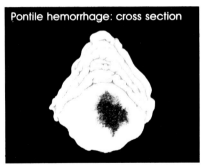

**Pontile hemorrhage: cross section**

In this representation of an image produced by CT scan, the dark area within the pons indicates bleeding.

large, a skull X-ray may show a shift of the pineal gland from the midline away from the hemorrhage. The patient's white blood cell count may be as high as 15,000 to 20,000 per cubic millimeter.

## CARING FOR YOUR STROKE PATIENT

After you know the location and size of your patient's hemorrhage, you can begin to devise a nursing-care plan. With a patient like Mr. Scanlon who suffered a cerebellar hemorrhage, the doctor may surgically evacuate or aspirate blood, to prevent compression of vital structures and further complications. So be ready to prepare your patient for surgery if the doctor chooses to take this approach.

---

*As a rule, surgery isn't an option for controlling a hemorrhage originating outside the cerebellum.*

---

The doctor may try to stop cerebellar bleeding by lowering blood pressure with adrenergic inhibitors. But since this approach has had little success, it remains controversial.

For a patient whose stroke originated in another part of the

brain, your nursing care will be mainly supportive and aimed at preventing increased intracranial pressure (see the chart on the following page for details).

If the patient's hemorrhage is small, chances are good that he'll make a complete recovery. His body will probably reabsorb the extravasated blood in time. Chances are, most brain tissue affected by the hemorrhage was displaced, rather than destroyed, and so will eventually function normally. To compensate for those tissue cells that were destroyed, nearby cells may begin to assume new functions.

If the patient's hemorrhage was massive, however, the prognosis is poor. Within a short time, the patient will probably die from brain stem compression.

# HEMORRHAGIC STROKE

## CARING FOR THE PATIENT WITH INCREASED INTRACRANIAL PRESSURE

Your patient with elevated intracranial pressure (ICP) requires special nursing care. Of course you'll monitor his condition frequently and document all your findings. In addition, you'll perform all nursing care measures as *carefully* and *gently* as possible to avoid further increasing his ICP.

Obviously, your patient with high ICP places great demands on your time and energy. But the expert and cautious care that you provide him could save his life. For a complete look at this special nursing care, refer to the chart below.

### NURSING ACTION

Maintain low $PCO_2$ and normal $PO_2$.
**Rationale**
• Low $PCO_2$ causes cerebral vasoconstriction, which helps reduce cerebral edema.
• Normal $PO_2$ prevents cerebral vasodilation.
**Additional considerations**
• Maintain a patent airway.
• Monitor arterial blood gases.
• Suction as necessary to clear secretions.

### NURSING ACTION

Maintain venous outflow from the brain.
**Rationale**
• Keeps capillary pressure down, which allows better absorption of cerebrospinal fluid (CSF)
• Prevents $CO_2$ and lactic acid buildup, which helps prevent cerebral vasodilation
**Additional considerations**
• Avoid prone or Trendelenburg position.
• Elevate head of bed 30°, or as ordered.
• Avoid neck flexion.
• Prevent jugular vein compression.

### NURSING ACTION

Maintain normal (or slightly below normal) body temperature.
**Rationale**
• Above-normal temperatures increase the brain's metabolic needs; slightly subnormal temperatures reduce metabolic needs. *Caution:* Shivering can increase ICP.
**Additional considerations**
• As ordered, give antipyretic drugs; use a hypothermia blanket, if ordered, to lower the patient's temperature.
• Give the patient chlorpromazine, if ordered, to control shivering.

### NURSING ACTION

Assist with withdrawal of CSF via ventricular catheter.
**Rationale**
• Decreases CSF volume, which reduces intracranial pressure
**Additional considerations**
• Assemble necessary equipment.
• Drain off CSF slowly while monitoring ICP (according to hospital policy and doctor's orders).
• Watch for any sudden change in neurologic status after procedure. A sudden drop in ICP may cause brain herniation.

### NURSING ACTION

Administer osmotic diuretics; for example, mannitol.
**Rationale**
• Reduces cerebral edema, shrinking intracranial contents
**Additional considerations**
• Check ampule or bottle closely for crystal formation before administering drug.
• Monitor fluids, electrolytes, and serum osmolality; osmotic diuretics may cause rapid dehydration.
• Closely watch elderly patients for signs of congestive heart failure.

### NURSING ACTION

Administer I.V. steroids, as ordered; for example, dexametha-
sone (Decadron). *Note:* This therapy is controversial.
**Rationale**
• Lowers sodium and water concentration in the brain, reducing cerebral edema
**Additional considerations**
• As ordered, give steroids with antacids or with cimetidine, orally or I.V., to prevent peptic ulcers.
• Watch for signs of GI bleeding.

### NURSING ACTION

Restrict fluids.
**Rationale**
• Prevents fluid overload, which reduces cerebral edema
**Additional considerations**
• Monitor fluids and electrolytes (including serum osmolality) closely. Keep accurate intake and output records, and maintain fluid restrictions, as ordered.
• Weigh the patient daily.

### NURSING ACTION

Induce coma by administering a barbiturate, as ordered; for example, phenobarbital.
**Rationale**
• Decreases cerebral metabolic rate; decreases cerebral blood flow
**Additional considerations**
• Monitor vital signs and ICP.
• Give barbiturates, as ordered.

### NURSING ACTION

Avoid increasing intrathoracic or intraabdominal pressure.
**Rationale**
• Added thoracic or abdominal pressure can spike ICP by increasing pressure on central veins.
**Additional considerations**
• Avoid Trendelenburg position.
• Prevent the Valsalva maneuver or similar practices, such as straining during bowel movements. Give stool softeners, as needed.
• Don't let your patient push against a footboard.
• Avoid extreme hip flexion.

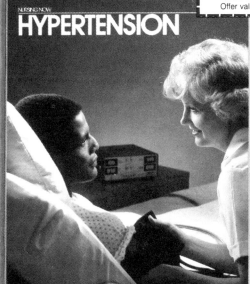
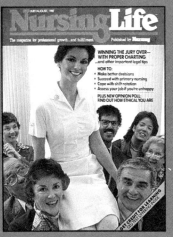

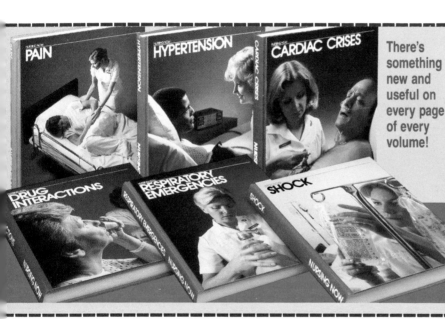
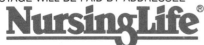

# RENOVASCULAR HYPERTENSION

## WHAT CAUSES RENOVASCULAR HYPERTENSION?

Renovascular hypertension, a type of secondary hypertension, is caused by decreased blood flow to one or both kidneys. Sensing decreased blood flow, the kidney releases renin and triggers the renin-angiotensin-aldosterone cycle. As you learned on pages 12 and 13, this cycle increases systemic blood pressure.

In most cases, decreased renal blood flow results from stenosis of the major renal arteries or their branches from one of two possible causes: atherosclerosis (usually where the renal artery joins the aorta) or fibromuscular dysplasia (which usually affects the middle and distal portions of renal vessels and may extend into the branches).

Atherosclerosis, the most common cause of renovascular hypertension, occurs most often in men above age 50. Fibromuscular dysplasia, by contrast, is more common in women under age 45. Although often bilateral, this condition usually affects the right kidney more severely than the left. Other, less common, causes for decreased renal blood flow include arteritis, anomalies of the renal arteries, embolus, trauma, tumor, and dissecting aneurysm.

The beaded appearance of the left renal artery is characteristic of fibromuscular dysplasia. The right renal artery is stenosed from atherosclerosis.

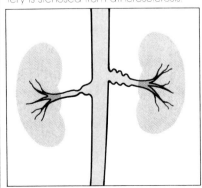

## RECOGNIZING SIGNS AND SYMPTOMS

Does your patient have renovascular hypertension? Be suspicious if his history reveals one or more of these factors:
• His hypertension is acute (or his previously mild hypertension has suddenly become severe).
• His condition hasn't responded to antihypertensive medication.
• He can't tolerate antihypertensive medication because of adverse reactions.
• He's younger than age 20 or older than age 50.

**Assessment.** On physical examination, the most revealing signs of renovascular hypertension are bruits. A high-pitched systolic bruit audible over the upper abdomen (and possibly radiating to either subcostal area) suggests fibromuscular dysplasia. Bruits audible over the abdomen and femoral or carotid arteries suggest atherosclerosis. But keep in mind that bruits are not always present in renovascular hypertension.

**Other findings.** In addition to bruits, your assessment findings may include one or more of the following:
• grade III or IV Keith-Wagoner-Barker funduscopic changes, including hemorrhages, exudates, and papilledema (see page 35 for details)
• unexplained hypokalemia
• polycythemia
• ptosis of the kidney, suggesting fibrous lesions.

*Note:* A patient with renovascular hypertension may experience symptoms characteristic of primary hypertension; for example, headaches, palpitations, anxiety, light-headedness, decreased tolerance of temperature extremes, and mental sluggishness.

## REVIEWING DIAGNOSTIC TESTS

If the doctor suspects that renal artery stenosis is responsible for your patient's hypertension, he'll take two steps. First, he'll order tests to help confirm the presence of stenosis. If stenosis is present, he'll then order more tests to determine if the stenosis is, in fact, responsible for the patient's hypertension. Why the second step? Because renal artery disease can *coexist* with primary hypertension without being its cause. Determining the relationship between the stenosis, if present, and the patient's hypertension helps the doctor choose appropriate treatment. *Note:* Some patients with significant renal disease never develop hypertension.

**The first step.** Initially, the doctor orders routine urine and blood analyses, including electrolyte, blood urea nitrogen, creatinine, and potassium studies. The results help him assess kidney function. Then, he'll order one or more of the following diagnostic tests. (Because a single test is rarely conclusive, expect him to order a combination of tests.) *Caution:* Most of the following tests require injection of radiopaque contrast dye. Be sure to inform the doctor and radiology department if the patient has an allergy to iodine or seafood.
• *Rapid-sequence intravenous pyelogram.* Intravenous injection of radiopaque dye permits visualization of the entire urinary tract on X-ray. This test (which is also called excretory urography) suggests unilateral stenosis if the dye's appearance is delayed on one side. For other significant findings, see page 37.
• *Saralasin test.* Saralasin, an angiotensin II antagonist, is rapidly infused I.V. while the patient's

CONTINUED ON PAGE 122

# RENOVASCULAR HYPERTENSION

## REVIEWING DIAGNOSTIC TESTS CONTINUED

blood pressure response is monitored. This relatively new test is positive for renin-dependent hypertension if diastolic pressure drops by 7 to 10 mm Hg (or more), or by more than 8%.

To enhance test results, the doctor may prepare the patient by restricting his sodium intake and ordering a diuretic to cause moderate sodium depletion. However, the value of this measure is controversial.

*Caution:* The patient may experience a sharp blood pressure increase after the infusion ends. Closely monitor his blood pressure during and after the infusion.

• *Radionuclide renography.* The patient receives an injection of hippuran that's tagged with a small amount of radioactive iodine. Then, counters are placed over his kidneys; they trace the progress of the radioactive isotopes through the kidneys and plot the information on a graph like the one shown on the opposite page. Because proper placement of the counters is essential, this test doesn't always provide reliable results.

• *Arteriography.* The most direct way to identify renal stenosis, arteriography is also the most reliable. But because it's an invasive procedure, this test also exposes the patient to more risks than noninvasive tests.

After inserting a catheter into the femoral artery, the doctor threads it into the aorta to the level of the second lumbar vertebra. Then he injects contrast dye through the catheter. The dye permits clear visualization of the renal arteries and its branches inside the kidney. If the patient has fibromuscular dysplasia, the test reveals characteristic lesions resembling a string of beads (see page 121).

**Further investigation.** Let's say the doctor has confirmed that your patient has renal artery stenosis. Now, he needs to determine whether the stenosis is responsible for your patient's hypertension. If it is, he may attempt to correct the stenosis surgically (if your patient is a surgical candidate). But if no relationship exists, and kidney function is adequate, he may treat the condition more conservatively.

If one of the previously mentioned tests reveals that a renal artery is more than 75% occluded, the doctor will probably assume that a significant relationship exists. But if the occlusion appears to be less than 75%, he may investigate further by ordering one or both of these tests:

*Renal vein renin sampling.* A catheter is inserted into the femoral vein and advanced into the inferior vena cava. Blood specimens are taken from each renal vein and from the inferior vena cava above and below the renal veins. Then the renin content of each specimen is analyzed. Any of the following results indicate significant renin output by the affected kidney, suggesting severe stenosis:

• a renal vein specimen with a renin concentration that's 50% greater than the renin concentration in a vena cava specimen; or, a concentration that's at least 50% greater than the average renin concentration in a mixed venous specimen
• a kidney-to-kidney ratio of 1.5 or more.

To enhance test results, the doctor may prepare the patient by ordering a low-sodium diet and diuretic therapy to cause sodium depletion. After the test, monitor the catheter insertion site

## READING A RENOGRAM

After your patient undergoes radionuclide renography, the doctor will receive a renogram that resembles the one shown here. The initial sharp rise in the dotted normal curve represents renal uptake of the radioactive isotope. Called the vascular phase, renal uptake usually follows within 30 to 45 seconds after isotope administration.

The tubular phase, which represents renal transit time, occurs next. This phase lasts up to 5 minutes and produces a curve that rises more gradually.

During the excretory phase, the isotope drains from the kidneys and the curve declines.

As shown in the other curve, when a renal artery is stenotic, the affected kidney takes up less of the isotope, and does so more slowly than normal. In addition, it excretes the isotope more slowly. When stenosis is present, therefore, the vascular phase curve is shorter and less steep than normal. Similarly, the excretory phase curve returns to the baseline more slowly than normal.

Key:
I = Vascular phase
II = Tubular phase
III = Excretory phase

for bleeding and other possible complications.

*Ureteral urine measurements* (also called a split function study). For this test, the patient receives a spinal anesthetic. One or both ureters are catheterized and successive urine specimens collected. The specimens are then analyzed for the concentration

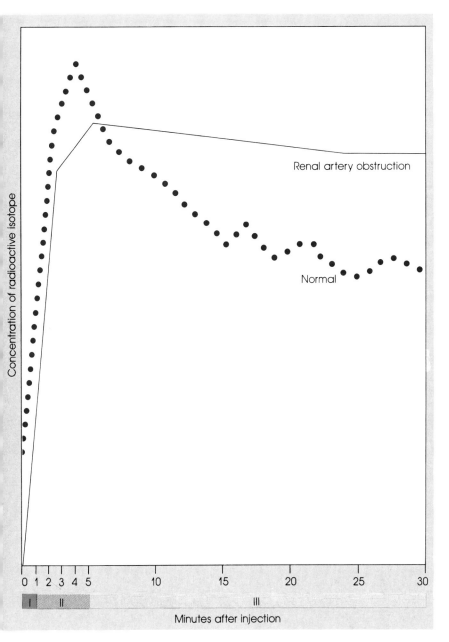

Concentration of radioactive isotope

Renal artery obstruction

Normal

0 1 2 3 4 5  10  15  20  25  30

I  II  III

Minutes after injection

## CARING FOR THE PATIENT UNDERGOING ARTERIOGRAPHY

If your patient's scheduled for renal arteriography, follow these guidelines for pre- and postop care.

**Before the procedure:**
• Explain the procedure to the patient. Prepare him for a possible flushing sensation or metallic taste when the contrast dye is injected.
• Ask him if he's allergic to iodine (or any iodine-containing foods, such as shellfish). If he is, inform the doctor.
• Instruct him not to eat for 8 hours before the test.
• Make sure the doctor's obtained a signed consent form.

**After the procedure:**
• Keep the patient flat in bed for 8 to 12 hours and on bed rest for up to 24 hours.
• Ask him to try to avoid straining during bowel movements, coughing, and sneezing.
• Check his vital signs every 15 minutes for 1 hour; then every 30 minutes for 2 hours, then hourly until they stabilize. Then, check them every 4 hours.
• If the doctor used a femoral insertion site, check the dorsalis pedis and popliteal pulses, and the color and temperature of the patient's lower legs every time you check vital signs. If the doctor used an axillary approach, check the radial pulse and the hand's temperature and color.
• For at least the first 8 hours, check the insertion site for hematoma or bleeding each time you check vital signs. Keep the pressure dressing in place.
• Be alert for lower back pain; it may indicate retroperitoneal bleeding.
• Maintain accurate fluid intake and output records until the patient is discharged. The contrast medium is nephrotoxic and also can cause osmotic diuresis.

of sodium and nonreabsorbable solutes, including creatinine and para-aminohippurate (PAH). A high concentration of these solutes, a low sodium concentration, and low urine output are all results that are consistent with severe stenosis.

*Note:* During the test, the doctor may administer I.V. infusions of 4% urea to produce adequate urine flow, and PAH to help determine the rate of PAH excretion.

Following the test, observe the patient for signs of these possible complications: ureteral obstruction from edema following traumatic catheter insertion, infection, or transient ureteral colic.

# SURGICAL TREATMENT

## TREATING THE PATIENT SURGICALLY

Depending on the results of diagnostic tests and the patient's blood pressure levels, the doctor may suggest one of these surgical procedures: renal artery bypass, endarterectomy, or nephrectomy.

His choice depends largely on the type and extent of the renal artery stenosis or occlusion. The following information briefly describes each of these surgical procedures.

**Renal artery bypass.** A graft, connected to the abdominal aorta and the renal artery, acts as a conduit enabling blood to flow from the aorta to the kidney, bypassing the obstructed area. Although synthetic grafts—usually

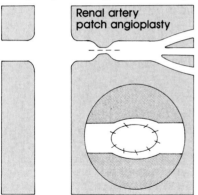

*Renal artery patch angioplasty*

After incising the artery's stenosed portion, the doctor removes the obstruction. He closes the incision with a patch graft (see circled illustration above).

Below, the doctor removes the renal artery's stenosed portion. Then, as shown in the circled illustration, he sutures the ends of the artery back together.

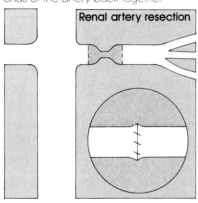

*Renal artery resection*

made of Dacron or Teflon—are sometimes used, a saphenous vein graft taken from the patient's thigh is preferred because it's compliant and more likely to remain patent.

During surgery, the doctor sutures one end of the bypass graft to the renal artery distal to the occlusion. Then he sutures the other end of the graft to the side of the aorta. (If the aorta is severely diseased, he can suture the graft to another artery, such as the hepatic or splenic artery.)

Since the bypass graft doesn't replace the renal artery, the kidney may continue to receive a blood supply if the graft ever occludes, permitting the kidney to survive until the occluded bypass graft is replaced. However, the part of the renal artery that was stenosed is likely to become completely occluded after the bypass, making the graft the kidney's only source of blood.

**Endarterectomy.** When the patient has an occlusion near the aorta, the doctor can open the aorta and surgically remove the blockage from within the lumen. If the stenosis is farther away from the aorta, he performs the endarterectomy through an incision in the renal artery. When he closes the incision, the doctor sutures a patch graft over it.

**Nephrectomy.** If all other surgical procedures fail, or if the patient has a severely atrophied kidney or obstructing lesions in the branch or small accessory arteries, the doctor may remove the affected kidney. A nephrectomy is always a last resort, used when drug therapy and other surgical procedures have failed.

*Note:* Other surgical options not discussed here include patch angioplasty and resection (dissection and end-to-end resection). Both procedures are shown at left.

## UNDERSTANDING PERCUTANEOUS TRANSLUMINAL ANGIOPLASTY

For one reason or another—perhaps because of the patient's age and physical condition—the doctor may decide that surgery isn't indicated for your patient. An older patient, for instance, may have atherosclerosis and other medical problems that make him a poor surgical risk. For such a patient, the doctor may suggest a nonsurgical, therapeutic procedure known as percutaneous transluminal angioplasty (PTA), or renal artery dilation. Similar to arteriography, PTA is an effective treatment for renovascular hypertension. But because the procedure isn't a cure, the problem may recur in the future.

**How PTA works.** The doctor inserts a double-lumen balloon catheter into the femoral artery. (If using the femoral artery is contraindicated, he may use an axillary approach instead.) Guided by fluoroscopy, he threads it through the aorta and into the renal artery. Next, he takes pressure readings on either side of the lesion to assess the amount of stenosis and the blood flow through the stenosed area. Then he positions the catheter and inflates the balloon, which dilates the stenotic artery. To prevent clotting, heparin is given by I.V. bolus.

After 30 to 60 seconds, the doctor deflates the balloon and takes blood pressure readings on either side of the lesion. If necessary, he may inflate and deflate the balloon several more times.

Throughout the procedure, renal arteriographs are taken. When the stenotic artery is sufficiently dilated, the doctor removes the catheter.

**Complications.** Possible complications of PTA include:
• bleeding, infection, false aneurysm, or thrombosis at the cathe-

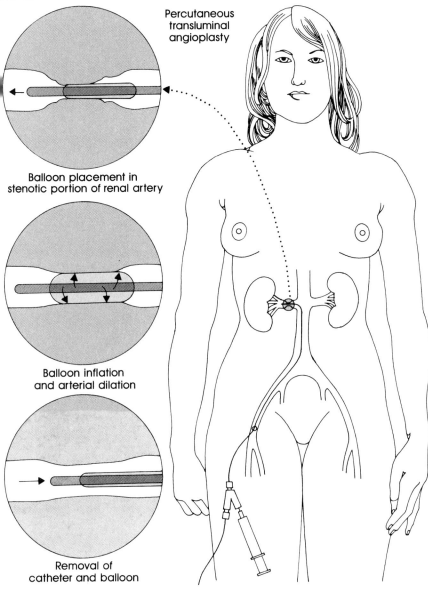

**Percutaneous transluminal angioplasty**

**Balloon placement in stenotic portion of renal artery**

**Balloon inflation and arterial dilation**

**Removal of catheter and balloon**

The illustration at upper right shows how a catheter is threaded into the renal artery from an insertion site in the femoral artery. The encircled close-ups at upper left illustrate the three-step procedure.

ter insertion site
• occlusion of distal arteries by clots or plaque dislodged during the procedure
• local damage to the renal artery wall during balloon inflation, causing cracking of the artery's intimal layer. Platelets may accumulate along these cracks, causing thrombosis. To minimize this risk, the doctor may order anticoagulant therapy after the procedure.

*Note:* For patient-care guidelines, review the information on page 122 relating to arteriography. Except for considerations pertaining to the contrast dye, care for the patient undergoing PTA is the same.

## POSTOPERATIVE CARE: SPECIAL CONSIDERATIONS

Following renal artery surgery, the patient will probably go to the intensive care unit. If you're responsible for him, you'll give the same routine care you'd provide for any postop patient. For example, you'll regularly monitor vital signs and fluid intake and output, as ordered, and you'll encourage regular deep breathing and coughing (see the teaching aid on page 116). Keep these special considerations in mind.

**Blood pressure.** Monitor the patient's blood pressure every 30 minutes to 1 hour. But don't expect it to drop to a normal level immediately following surgery. His blood pressure may remain slightly above the baseline level or even increase further for as long as 48 hours after surgery. (In these circumstances, the doctor may order a vasodilator, such as nitroprusside sodium, for blood pressure control. Closely monitor the patient for hypotension.)

Following surgery, blood pressure improves in about 90% of all patients who undergo renal artery surgery to correct renovascular hypertension. And, in some cases, the surgery cures the hypertension. But even when surgery is successful, blood pressure usually doesn't stabilize at a normal level for several weeks to months after surgery.

**Urine output.** When you monitor urine output, expect an increase in urine volume. But watch for *excessive* diuresis, which could cause hypovolemia and electrolyte imbalance. Document intake and output meticulously.

**Complications.** Your patient with renovascular hypertension is likely to have arteriosclerosis. If so, he's at a greater risk of myocardial infarction and other cardiovascular complications after surgery.

# PEDIATRICS

## WHEN YOUR PATIENT IS A CHILD

A child is considered hypertensive only if his blood pressure is significantly and consistently higher than 95% of children in his age-group (see the charts on page 127 for details). Because pediatric hypertension is unusual, you may rarely encounter it. So even if you're confident about your ability to care for a hypertensive adult, you may feel somewhat uncertain about how to help a child.

And treating a child *is* different than treating an adult in many ways. Standard treatment regimens are well established for managing hypertension in an adult, but exactly how—and when—to treat a hypertensive child is controversial. Read the next few pages for guidelines to follow when caring for this special patient.

## TAKING A CHILD'S BLOOD PRESSURE: A SPECIAL CHALLENGE

Taking a child's blood pressure is sometimes easier said than done. For one thing, the child may be anxious and uncooperative, making an accurate reading difficult to obtain. Read what follows for some tips to make the task easier—for you *and* your patient.

**Encouraging cooperation.** For best results, always try to take blood pressure readings when your patient's calm and relaxed. But a pediatric patient may not be so accommodating. You may have to contend with a child who's restless, anxious, or combative. Take time to establish rapport with the child and gain his confidence. Show him the blood pressure equipment; then, take his parent's blood pressure to show him that the procedure won't hurt. If he seems uncom-

fortable or frightened by lying on the examining table, allow him to sit up.

**Taking readings.** A child's blood pressure fluctuates more than an adult's. So, to get an accurate blood pressure measurement, you'll need to take at least three readings at different times.

Some controversy exists over which Korotkoff phase to document as the diastolic measurement—the muffled 4th phase, which may provide a false-high reading, or the hard-to-detect 5th phase, which may provide a false-low reading. The best you can do is to document both phases; for example, 130/76/62 (I/IV/V).

*Note:* When taking a reading, don't press the stethoscope's diaphragm too hard against the antecubital fossa. You may distort the Korotkoff sounds.

## SELECTING THE PROPER BLOOD PRESSURE CUFF

Which cuff size is appropriate for your pediatric patient? Use the following chart as a guide.

*Important:* If your patient's

unusually large or small for his age-group, select a cuff that's appropriate for his *size*, not his age.

| AGE CATEGORY | CUFF WIDTH | CUFF LENGTH |
|---|---|---|
| Newborn | 2.5 to 4.0 cm | 5.0 to 10.0 cm |
| Infant | 6.0 to 8.0 cm | 12.0 to 13.5 cm |
| Child | 9.0 to 10.0 cm | 17.0 to 22.5 cm |
| Adult | 12.0 to 13.0 cm | 22.0 to 23.5 cm |

Source: *Report of the Task Force on Blood Pressure Control in Children,* The National Heart, Lung, and Blood Institute (NHLBI), 1977.

## USING BLOOD PRESSURE GRIDS

When diagnosing pediatric hypertension, the doctor may use the blood pressure grids shown at right. These grids, which are available from the High Blood Pressure Information Center, enable him to compare the child's blood pressure with normal blood pressures for the child's age-group and sex. Hypertension may be present if three or four consecutive blood pressure readings exceed the 95th percentile for the child's age and sex.

For an accurate comparison, always take the patient's blood pressure reading in his right arm, while he's sitting. The grids were developed from blood pressure measurements taken under these circumstances.

*Note:* On the average, girls have higher blood pressures than boys until puberty. After puberty, the trend reverses.

## SELECTING THE PROPER BLOOD PRESSURE METHOD

In addition to determining cuff size, your pediatric patient's age and size influence the method you use to take his blood pressure. Choose from among these three noninvasive alternatives.

**The ultrasound method.** When examining a newborn (either premature or full-term), use an ultrasound Doppler monitor. More accurate than the sphygmomanometer, the ultrasound monitor picks up frequency changes produced by blood flow variations and either amplifies the sounds or represents them on an oscilloscope. This gives you an accurate systolic pressure reading and a good estimate of diastolic pressure in most infants.

**The flush method.** When examining an infant less than age 1, use the flush method if the Doppler

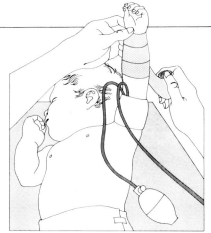

**Using the flush method**
The flush method is one way to take an infant's blood pressure accurately.

isn't available. Here's how.
• Apply a proper-size blood pressure cuff.
• Elevate the infant's arm or thigh (either will do since the arm and thigh pressure of a child this age are equal).
• Wrap an elastic bandage from

his wrist to his elbow or from his ankle to his knee.
• Wait until his hand (or foot) becomes pale; then, inflate the blood pressure cuff.
• Unwrap and lower the limb, and begin deflating the cuff. Note the pressure reading when the hand or foot flushes from blood return.

This approximate reading isn't the infant's systolic or diastolic pressure, but rather his *mean* arterial blood pressure. In infants this age, the upper limit of normal flush pressure is approximately 80 mm Hg.

**The conventional method.** When examining a child who's age 3 or older, use a conventional blood pressure cuff and sphygmomanometer. Since a child's Korotkoff sounds are harder to hear than an adult's, remember to take the reading in a quiet setting.

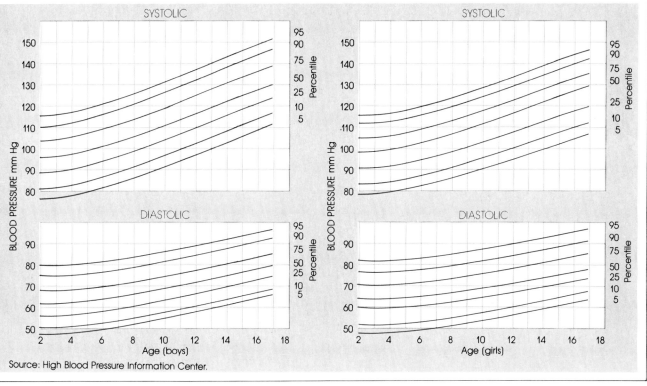

Source: High Blood Pressure Information Center.

# PEDIATRICS

## ASSESSING A CHILD FOR HYPERTENSION

Like many hypertensive adults, a child with hypertension may be asymptomatic. That's why a thorough health history is especially important. If your patient's blood pressure reading is high, take the time to investigate further.

**Assessment findings.** When taking the child's health history, ask him (or his parent) if he ever experiences recurring headaches (especially throbbing frontal headaches), dizziness, fatigue, or nosebleeds. Although they may not be significant, all these signs and symptoms sometimes accompany hypertension. For example, about one third of all hypertensive children experience headaches.

Also note any factors that might predispose the child to hypertension; for example, obesity, high sodium intake, or a family history of hypertension.

**Identifying the cause.** Before puberty, secondary hypertension is far more common than primary hypertension. The most common secondary causes are renal disease, cardiac disease, and adrenal disorders. Depending on the specific cause, the child may exhibit signs of congestive heart failure, decreased femoral pulses, café-au-lait spots, or abdominal or flank bruits. Read the chart at right for more information about some common causes of secondary hypertension in children and the characteristic signs and symptoms they produce.

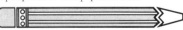

SPECIAL NOTE: When you take a health history, ask the child's parent if the child has taken any cold remedies lately. Many cold remedies contain ephedrine, a drug that can elevate blood pressure.

## IDENTIFYING SECONDARY HYPERTENSION

If you suspect that your pediatric patient has secondary hypertension, can you identify the most likely cause? Read the following chart for guidance.

*Note:* Pheochromocytoma is a possible cause of pediatric hypertension that's not mentioned here. For details on this condition, review pages 112 to 117.

### COARCTATION OF THE AORTA (ABDOMINAL)

**History**
• Sudden attacks of abdominal pain

**Assessment findings**
• Severely high blood pressure (180/120 mm Hg or higher)
• Decreased or absent femoral pulses
• Dyspnea
• Flank or abdominal bruits
• Decreased circulation in legs and feet
• Fatigue on exertion
• Convulsions (rare)

**Test results**
• Chest X-ray reveals mild to moderate heart enlargement and rib-notching.
• Arteriogram reveals coarctation of aorta.
• Cardiac catheterization may reveal left-to-right shunts and other congenital abnormalities.

### COARCTATION OF THE AORTA (THORACIC)

Thoracic and abdominal coarctation of the aorta are the most common cardiac-related causes of pediatric hypertension.

**History**
• Feeding problems

**Assessment findings**
• Signs and symptoms of congestive heart failure; for example, dyspnea, pulmonary edema, tachypnea, tachycardia, enlarged heart, gallop rhythm, rales, pallor, enlarged liver
• Inadequate weight gain
• Lethargy

**Test results**
• Chest X-ray reveals mild to moderate heart enlargement and rib-notching.
• Arteriogram reveals coarctation of aorta.
• Cardiac catheterization may reveal left-to-right shunts and other congenital abnormalities.

### ACUTE POSTSTREPTOCOCCAL GLOMERULONEPHRITIS

Most prevalent cause of renovascular hypertension in pediatric patients

**History**
• Upper respiratory tract or skin infection within past 5 weeks
• Rapid weight gain and decreased urine output

**Assessment findings**
• Malaise
• Anorexia
• Mild headaches
• Edema
• Oliguria
• Proteinuria
• Hematuria
• Uremia
• Venous dilation on funduscopy
• Seizures, congestive heart failure, or acute renal failure in severe cases

**Test results**
• Blood tests reveal elevated titers of streptozyme or antistreptolysin, decreased $C_3$ and $C_4$ components of complement assay, elevated creatinine and blood urea nitrogen (BUN) levels; and increased potassium level (if child is anuric).
• Evidence of streptococcal infection apparent in blood, urine, or other culture.

### RENOVASCULAR DISEASE

**History**
• Headaches
• Abdominal or flank trauma
• Hematuria
• Slow growth rate
*Note:* The following may be seen if the patient also has adrenal in-

volvement: signs and symptoms of aldosteronism (for example, polyuria, polydyspnea, and hypokalemia) and a family history of neurofibromatosis.

**Assessment findings**
• Abdominal or flank bruits
• In adrenal involvement, café-au-lait spots; signs and symptoms of neurofibromatosis (for example, cutaneous and subcutaneous neurofibromas, hyperpigmentation, and congenital malformations)

**Test results**
• Renal vein renin measurement reveals elevated renin levels.
• Intravenous pyelogram (IVP) reveals functional differences between the kidneys.

## UNILATERAL RENAL PARENCHYMAL DISEASE

**History**
• Recurring urinary tract infection
• Fever
• Abdominal or flank trauma

**Assessment findings**
• Enlarged kidney
• Tenderness around the costovertebral angle in acute cases
• Hematuria possible

**Test results**
• Renal vein renin measurement reveals elevated renin levels.
• Urinalysis may reveal proteinuria.
• Arteriogram may reveal renal artery stenosis.
• IVP may reveal functional differences between the kidneys.

## DRUG THERAPY: PEDIATRIC CONSIDERATIONS

To treat a hypertensive child, the doctor will first take a conservative, nonpharmacologic approach by prescribing diet changes, weight reduction (if necessary), and regular exercise. But if these measures fail to control the child's condition, he'll probably order drug therapy, taking the same stepped-care approach he'd use for an adult patient. Of course, he'll adjust therapy according to the child's age and size.

The following chart details pediatric considerations for the most commonly prescribed drugs in Steps 1 through 3 of the stepped-care regimen. Because of their potency, Step 4 drugs are rarely prescribed for children.

### STEP 1: DIURETICS
#### Chlorothiazide

**Pediatric dosage**
Children under age 6 months: 30 mg/kg P.O. daily in two divided doses. Children over age 6 months: 20 mg/kg P.O. daily in divided doses.

**Possible adverse reactions**
Volume depletion and dehydration, hypokalemia (serum potassium concentration less than 3.5 mEq/liter), hyperuricemia, hypercalcemia, hyperglycemia, thrombocytopenia

#### Hydrochlorothiazide

**Pediatric dosage**
Children under age 6 months: up to 3.3 mg/kg P.O. daily, b.i.d. Children over age 6 months: 2.2 mg/kg P.O. daily, b.i.d.

**Possible adverse reactions**
Volume depletion and dehydration, hypokalemia (serum potassium concentration less than 3.5 mEq/liter), hyperuricemia, hypercalcemia, hyperglycemia

#### Furosemide

**Pediatric dosage**
2 mg/kg daily; increase by 1 to 2 mg/kg in 6 to 8 hours, if needed. Titrate carefully up to 6 mg/kg daily, if needed.

**Possible adverse reactions**
Volume depletion and dehydration, abdominal pain, hypokalemia, asymptomatic hyperuricemia, hypocalcemia, hypoglycemia.

*Important:* Avoid giving a child this drug by a parenteral route, if possible.

### STEP 2: ADRENERGIC INHIBITORS
#### Methyldopa

**Pediatric dosage**
Initially, 10 mg/kg daily P.O. in three to four divided doses; not to exceed 250 mg/dose. Increase daily dosage until desired response occurs. Maximum daily dosage: 65 mg/kg.

**Possible adverse reactions**
Hemolytic anemia, drowsiness, fatigue, irritability or emotional lability, diarrhea, orthostatic hypotension

### STEP 3: VASODILATORS
#### Hydralazine hydrochloride

**Pediatric dosage**
Initially, 0.75 mg/kg P.O. daily in four to six divided doses. May increase gradually to 10 times this dosage, if necessary.

**Possible adverse reactions**
Headache, tachycardia, nausea, vomiting, lupus erythematosus-like syndrome (rare)

# GERIATRICS

## CARING FOR THE GERIATRIC PATIENT: HOW AGE MAKES A DIFFERENCE

Planning your nursing care may be a bit more involved for a hypertensive geriatric patient than for a younger adult. Why? Because the aging process plays a major role in an elderly patient's response to therapy—especially drug therapy. Because his vascular, gastrointestinal, and autonomic nervous systems are altered by the aging process, his response to drug therapy may be difficult to predict. As a result, adverse reactions are more likely—and some are potentially fatal.

To minimize risk, the doctor will probably take a conservative approach when prescribing therapy. If the patient is already taking medications for other medical conditions that may occur among the elderly (for example, congestive heart failure), the addition of antihypertensive drugs increases the risk of adverse reactions. And, because the patient now has more drugs to remember to take, compliance may decline.

Besides the physiologic changes that occur in an elderly patient, also consider his economic status. If he's living on a fixed income, he may be unable to afford prescribed drugs and a nutritious daily diet.

For these reasons and more, your care plan must be based on a complete and thorough patient assessment that takes into account the patient's established life-style and his continued well-being. On these two pages, we'll tell you how to assess, care for, and deal with the special problems of hypertension in the older adult.

## TYPES OF GERIATRIC HYPERTENSION

Hypertension affects geriatric patients in much the same way it affects younger patients. Consider these points:
• Geriatric hypertension is asymptomatic; most elderly patients learn they're hypertensive only after seeking treatment for another disorder.
• Hypotension among geriatric patients increases the risk of cardiovascular and kidney disease. If an elderly patient already has arteriosclerosis or congestive heart failure, hypertension may worsen the condition.

Unlike hypertension among younger patients, however, an acceptable systolic pressure for an elderly patient can be as high as 160 mm Hg. Diastolic and systolic blood pressures are normally higher for elderly adults than for younger adults.

**Systolic hypertension** (systolic pressure 160 mm Hg or greater with a diastolic pressure less than 90 mm Hg). This is the most common type of geriatric hypertension. It occurs as the aorta and major arteries become stiffer from aging and arteriosclerosis. Depending on the patient's condition, including the degree of target organ damage (if any), the doctor may decide against treatment. Or, he may prescribe drug therapy.

**Diastolic hypertension** (diastolic pressure of 90 mm Hg or greater). This type of hypertension is usually accompanied by renal disease. Antihypertensive drug therapy is recommended for all forms of diastolic hypertension: mild (96 to 105 mm Hg), moderate (106 to 120 mm Hg), and severe (above 120 mm Hg).

## ASSESSING THE ELDERLY PATIENT

Assess your elderly patient as you would a younger patient: with a health history, physical examination, and laboratory evaluation, as ordered. Keep these special considerations in mind during your assessment:
• When measuring an elderly patient's blood pressure, be sure to inflate the blood pressure cuff 20 to 30 mm Hg above the patient's palpatory systolic pressure to assure an accurate systolic reading.
• Take blood pressure readings with the patient in at least two positions: lying and standing, or sitting and standing. The readings will alert you to postural changes and help you anticipate possible complications of antihypertensive drug therapy.
• Always obtain baseline blood pressure readings in both arms and note any differences.
• Be aware that complicated diagnostic tests, such as renal scan and radiographic aortography, are usually unwarranted since drug therapy, as opposed to surgery, offers the best prognosis for the elderly patient. Likewise, tests for serum renin and aldosterone levels are usually unnecessary.
• Be sure to rule out hyperthyroidism, arteriovenous fistula, Paget's disease, and severe anemia as possible causes of the patient's increased blood pressure.

## TREATING GERIATRIC HYPERTENSION

The question of when to start drug therapy for a geriatric patient remains controversial. Some doctors recommend drug therapy for elderly patients with blood pressures greater than 160/90 mm Hg; others recommend a low-salt diet, weight loss, and relaxation measures for patients with systolic pressures ranging from 180 to 200 mm Hg. However, under these circumstances, drug therapy is always indicated:
• diastolic pressure greater than 105 mm Hg for three consecutive readings
• systolic pressure greater than 200 mm Hg for three consecutive readings
• extensive target organ damage
• rising hypertension alone or combined with congestive heart failure, renal failure, cerebral hemorrhage, angina pectoris, or aortic aneurysm.

Whenever drug therapy is prescribed, dosage should be low enough to allow for a gradual blood pressure drop, which prevents hypotension, drowsiness, restlessness, and decreased renal blood flow. For most geriatric patients, drug therapy starts with a minimum, once-daily dose of an oral, thiazide-type diuretic (a Step 1 drug). However, if the patient shows signs of renal impairment or congestive heart failure (or has a history of these problems), the doctor may substitute another diuretic, such as furosemide.

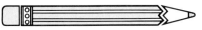

SPECIAL NOTE: Since the potassium loss created by diuretic therapy can lead to hypokalemia, carefully assess the patient's diet to make sure it contains enough high-potassium foods, such as bananas and fresh orange juice.

If the patient is taking a diuretic and digitalis, he may need a potassium supplement. If present, hypokalemia increases the risk of digitalis toxicity.

If a diuretic doesn't sufficiently reduce the patient's blood pressure in 4 to 6 weeks, the doctor may add a Step 2 adrenergic inhibitor. However, this drug type isn't recommended for most elderly hypertensive patients because drug effects are unpredictable and may lead to dangerous blood pressure fluctuations. For the same reason, Step 3 and Step 4 drugs are rarely prescribed.

## HOW AGING AFFECTS ANTIHYPERTENSIVE DRUG ACTION

Depending on the physiologic changes your patient has undergone, medications may act in unpredictable and sometimes undesirable ways. Keep the following information in mind when administering antihypertensive drug therapy to a geriatric patient.

### IF YOUR PATIENT HAS: DECREASED CARDIAC OUTPUT

**And you administer these drugs:**
All antihypertensive medications

**Expect these results:**
• Delayed onset of medication effect
• Medication effect prolonged, because the medication stays in the circulation longer

### IF YOUR PATIENT HAS: ALTERED BODY WEIGHT OR COMPOSITION

**And you administer these drugs:**
All antihypertensive medications

**Expect this result:**
• Unpredictable distribution and action of medication

### IF YOUR PATIENT HAS: DECREASED LIVER FUNCTION

**And you administer this drug:**
Propranolol hydrochloride

**Expect this result:**
• Increased risk of toxicity from slower metabolism of medication

### IF YOUR PATIENT HAS: DECREASED RENAL FUNCTION

**And you administer these drugs:**
Furosemide, metolazone, thiazides, diazoxide, guanethidine sulfate, methyldopa, chlorthalidone

**Expect this result:**
• Medication excretion reduced

### IF YOUR PATIENT HAS: DECREASED SERUM ALBUMIN

**And you administer these drugs:**
Propranolol hydrochloride, hydralazine, prazosin hydrochloride, chlorthalidone, furosemide, spironolactone

**Expect these results:**
• Decreased protein for binding
• Increased serum concentration of medication, which heightens medication effect

# REFERENCES AND ACKNOWLEDGMENTS

## Books

Beeson, Paul B., et al., ed. *Cecil Textbook of Medicine,* 16th ed. Philadelphia: W.B. Saunders Co., 1982.

Blackburn, Henry. "Risk Factors and Cardiovascular Disease," in *The American Heart Association Heartbook.* New York: E.P. Dutton, 1980.

Davis, James O., et al., eds. *Hypertension: Mechanisms, Diagnosis, & Management.* New York: HP Publishing Company, Inc., 1977.

*Drugs.* Nurses Reference Library. Springhouse, Pa.: Springhouse Corporation, 1983.

Gross, Franz, and Robertson, J. I. S., eds. *Arterial Hypertension.* London: Pitman Books Ltd., 1979.

Guyton, Arthur C. *Textbook of Medical Physiology,* 6th ed. Philadelphia: W. B. Saunders Co., 1982.

Jenkins, C. David. "Behavioral Risk Factors," in *The American Heart Association Heartbook.* New York: E. P. Dutton, 1980.

Kaplan, N. *Clinical Hypertension,* 3rd ed. Baltimore: Williams & Wilkins Co., 1982.

Kochar, Mahendr, and Daniels, Lynda M. *Hypertension Control for Nurses and Other Health Professionals.* St. Louis: C. V. Mosby Co., 1978.

Krupp, Marcus A., and Chatton, Milton J., eds. *Current Medical Diagnosis and Treatment 1981.* Los Altos, Calif.: Lange Medical Pubns., 1981.

McMahon, F. G. *Management of Essential Hypertension.* New York: Futura Publishing Company, Inc., 1978.

Phillips, Raymond E. *Cardiovascular Therapy: A Systematic Approach,* Vol. I, 2nd ed. Philadelphia: W. B. Saunders Co., 1979.

Ramsey, J. M. *Basic Pathophysiology: Modern Stress and the Disease Process.* Menlo Park, Calif.: Addison-Wesley Publishing Co., 1982.

Sabiston, David C., Jr., ed. *Davis-Christopher Textbook of Surgery: The Biological Basis of Modern Surgical Practice,* 12th ed. Philadelphia: W. B. Saunders Co., 1981.

Schwartz, S. I., ed. *Principles of Surgery.* New York: McGraw-Hill Book Co., 1979.

## Periodicals and pamphlets

Andrews, G., et al. "Hypertension: Comparison of Drug and Nondrug Treatments," *British Medical Journal* 284:1523-1526, 1982.

Arkwright, P. D. "Effects of Alcohol Use and Other Aspects of Lifestyle on Blood Pressure Levels and Prevalence of Hypertension in a Working Population," *Circulation* 66:60-66, 1982.

Bananno, J., and Lies, J. E. "Effects of Physical Training on Coronary Risk Factors," *The American Journal of Cardiology* 33:760-764, 1974.

Berchtold, Peter, et al. "Obesity and Hypertension: Cardiovascular Response to Weight Reduction," *Hypertension* 4:50-54, 1982.

Bullen, M. U. "What Patients with Hypertension Should Know About Their Medication," *Drugs* 19:373-379, 1980.

Chobanian, Aram. "Hypertension," *Clinical Symposia* 34(5), 1982.

Fink, Janis W. "The Challenge of High Blood Pressure Control," *Nursing Clinics of North America* 16:301-308, 1981.

Fletcher, Gerald. "Exercise and Coronary Risk Factor Modification in the Management of Atherosclerosis," *Heart and Lung* 10:811-813, 1981.

Foster, S., and Kousch, D. C. "Adherence to Therapy in Hypertensive Patients," *Nursing Clinics of North America* 16:331, June 1981.

Foster, S., and Kousch, D. C. "Promoting Patient Adherence," *American Journal of Nursing* 78(5):829-832, 1978.

Foster, S. B., et al. "Influence of Side Effects of Antihypertensive Medications on Patient Behavior," *Cardiovascular Nursing* 14(2):9-14, 1978.

Friedman, G. D., et al. "Alcohol, Tobacco, and Hypertension," *Hypertension,* Supplement III 4:143-150.

Froelicher, V. F. "Exercise and the Prevention of Coronary Atherosclerotic Heart Disease," *Cardiovascular Clinics* 9(3):13-23, 1978.

Geddes, L. A., and Whistler, J. J. "The Error in Indirect Blood Pressure Measurement with the Incorrect Size of Cuff," *American Heart Journal* 96:4-8, 1978.

Hackett, T. P., and Cassem, N. H. *Coronary Care: Patient Psychology,* Dallas: American Heart Association, 1975.

Haddy, F. J. "Mechanism, Prevention and Therapy of Sodium-Dependent Hypertension," *American Journal of Medicine* 69:746-755, 1980.

Healton, E., et al. "Hypertensive Encephalopathy and the Neurologic Manifestations of Malignant Hypertension," *Neurology* 32:127, February 1982.

*Heart Facts.* Dallas: American Heart Association, 1979.

Hill, M. "Hypertension: What Can Go Wrong When You Measure Blood Pressure?" *American Journal of Nursing* 80:942, May 1980.

Hill, Martha N., and McCombs, Nova Jean, eds. "Hypertension," *Nursing Clinics of North America* 16(2), June 1981.

Hovell, M. F. "The Experimental Evidence for Weight-Loss Treatment of Essential Hypertension: A Critical Review," *American Journal of Public Health* 72:359-368, 1982.

Kannel, William B., and Dawber, Thomas R. "Contributors to Coronary Risks: Ten Years Later," *Heart and Lung* 11:60-64, 1982.

Kannel, William B., et al. "The relation of Adiposity to Blood Pressure on Development of Hypertension (The Framingham Study)," *Annals of Internal Medicine* 67:48-59, 1967.

Kirkendall, William, et al. "Recommendations for Human Blood Pressure Determination by Sphygmomanometers from the Subcommittee of the American Heart Association Postgraduate Education Committee," *Circulation* 62:1146A, 1980.

Lieberman, Ellin. "Hypertension in Childhood and Adolescence," *Clinical Symposia* 30(3), 1978.

Milhorn, H. T. "Cardiovascular Fitness," *American Family Physician* 26:163-169, 1982.

"Multiple Risk Factor Intervention Trial, Risk Factor Changes and Mortality Results," *Journal of the American Medical Association* '248:1465-1501, 1982.

"1980 Report of The Joint National Committee on Detection, Evaluation, and Treatment of High Blood Pressure," *Archives of Internal Medicine* 140:1280-1285, 1980.

*Nursing Education in High Blood Pressure Control.* U.S. Department of Health, Education, and Welfare, NIH Publication 76-1052, 1976.

Perlman, Lawrence V., et al. "Accuracy of Sphygmomanometers in Hospital Practice," *Archives of Internal Medicine* 125:1000-1003, 1970.

"Report of the Task Force on Blood Pressure Control in Children," *Pediatrics,* Supplement 59(5):797-820, 1977.

Richmond, Julius B., and Levy, Robert I. *Exercise and Your Heart.* U.S. Department of Health and Human Services, NIH Publication #81-1677, 1981.

Richter, J. M., and Sloan, R. "Stress. The Relaxation Technique," *American Journal of Nursing* 79:1960-1962, 1979.

Segal, J. "Hypertensive Emergencies: Practical Approach to Treatment," *Postgraduate Medicine* 68:107, August 1980.

Vidt, D. "Malignant Hypertension and the Hypertensive Crisis: Handling All Hazards," *Modern Medicine* 50:138, May 1982.

Wheeler, Linda, and Jones, Mary Brewer. "Pregnancy-Induced Hypertension," *JOGN Nursing* 10(3):212-232, June 1981.

Willis, Susan E., et al. "Hypertension in Pregnancy," *American Journal of Nursing* 82(5):791-822, May 1982.

**We'd like to thank the following companies for their help with this book:**

CRITIKON, INC.
Chadds Ford, Pa.

METROPOLITAN LIFE INSURANCE COMPANY
New York

WELCH ALLYN, INC.
Skaneateles Falls, N.Y.

**We'd also like to thank the staffs of:**

ABINGTON MEMORIAL HOSPITAL
Abington, Pa.
Marc S. Lapayowker, MD
Chairman, Department of Radiology

AMERICAN HEART ASSOCIATION
Dallas

GRAND VIEW HOSPITAL
Sellersville, Pa.
Arlene G. Feltstein, RN
Chief I.V. Therapist

L'AEROBICS
North Wales, Pa.
Roni Collier
Instructor

LANSDALE MEDICAL GROUP
Lansdale, Pa.
William R. Truscott, MD

MT. SINAI MEDICAL CENTER
Milwaukee
Michael L. Pollock, PhD
Director of Cardiac Rehabilitation Program

NATIONAL INSTITUTE OF HEALTH—NATIONAL HEART, LUNG, AND BLOOD INSTITUTE
Bethesda, Md.

UNIVERSITY OF NORTH CAROLINA
Chapel Hill
Joseph H. Perlmutt, PhD
Professor of Physiology, School of Medicine

UNIVERSITY OF WASHINGTON
Seattle
Anne Loustau, RN, PhD
Assistant Professor, School of Nursing

VETERANS ADMINISTRATION MEDICAL CENTER
Seattle
Barbara J. Blair, RNC, ANP, MN
Nurse Practitioner

WILLS EYE HOSPITAL
Philadelphia
Heather Boyd-Monk, RN, SRN, BSN
Educational Coordinator, Nursing Education

Chart on page 53 reprinted with permission from Barbara J. Blair, RNC, ANP, MN, and Anne Loustau, RN, PhD, "A Key to Compliance," *Nursing81,* 11(2), February 1981.

# INDEX

# INDEX

classifying preeclampsia, 103
critical questions, 106
diet, 107
drug therapy, 109
eclampsia care, 110-111
patient care for severe pre-
    eclampsia, 109
postpartum care, 111
predicting, 103
recognizing, 106
understanding, 100-102
urine testing, 107
Primary hypertension
definition of, 14
factors contributing to, 14
Propranolol hydrochloride, 80-81
Prostaglandins, 13
Pseudoaldosteronism, definition of, 19
Pyelonephritis, definition of, 18-19

Risk factors, 22
Roll-over test, 103

preparing the patient for, 88
reviewing Step 4 drugs, 87
urine protein test, 89
Stethoscope, equipment check, 24
Stress
biofeedback, 66
deep relaxation exercises, 65
understanding, 64-65